Aligning | Life

THE STINSON WELLNESS MODEL

Who are your heroes? What have they modeled that you would like to be true of your life? How would your life be different if you were living closer to your ideals than you are now?

In the back of all our minds are dreams, ideals, and expectations. When asked what it means to live well, we, to some extent, compare our realities with our ideals. The problem is that many of us dream but fail to develop realistic strategies that help turn dreams into reality and consequently find ourselves stuck in a rut with no idea how to move forward. Which dreams of yours would be realized if your life was aligned with your inner aspirations?

ALIGNING LIFE

The Stinson Wellness Model

David D. Stinson

Published by Stinson Education
Abbotsford, BC, Canada

Aligning Life: The Stinson Wellness Model
Second Edition
by David D. Stinson, M.Ed.

Copyright © 2015 by David D. Stinson

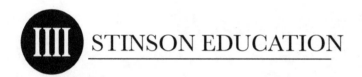 STINSON EDUCATION

Published by Stinson Education, Abbotsford, BC, Canada
www.stinsoneducation.com
stinsoneducation@gmail.com

Cover picture: Mike Stinson
Design: Tim Stinson
Editing: Andrea Slamaj, Faith Richardson

Originally published by Fox Song Books, Ferndale, WA, USA
Copyright 2013
Library of Congress Control Number: 2013955078

ISBN 978-0-9938478-0-6 (Second Edition)

Printed in Canada

This book is dedicated ...

To Becky, the love of my life, who has supported and encouraged me in the journey.

To Mike, Tim, and Matt. Hopefully you will find some wisdom herein.

To Dave, Michele, Faith, Mark, and many others who have influenced the development of this book.

Acknowledgments

Nothing like this happens in a vacuum. Many people and conversations have helped clarify my thoughts in places such as the carpool, staff meetings, road trips, church, the office, classes, and conferences. If you have been my friend in the last ten years, you have likely listened to me explain the wellness model and have offered constructive advice. In particular, the collegiality, insights, and support from colleagues at Trinity Western University have been amazing. It is a wonderful place to work and grow. So to all my friends and colleagues, thank you. You have been a significant part of the creation of this book.

Figures

Contents

Aligning|Life

PROLOGUE

I used to think good people automatically live well. In fact, I thought a lot of things happened automatically. I believed, for example, that wisdom and maturity increased with age and I would have my life figured out when I had a good career. While change and aging are constants, living well during different stages of life takes a mix of risk and intentionality.

What does wellness look like? And how does it feel? Is wellness when life is going our way, or can we live well during the tough times too? What aspects of life are included in the idea of wellness? We will discuss this further, later in the book, but it is important to understand that living well is related to how we live every part of our lives. While some aspects of life are more critical than others, living well includes all of them. As I write this book, I am doing so at the expense of other important things. Tasks need my attention. There is work I should do on the house and cars. Relationships also need attention. I have not had as much time to devote to good friends, as I would like. I have had fewer deep conversations with my wife and kids because we have not had as much time to spend together. Adding the writing of this book to the pressure of my busy job, the desire to be a good husband and father along with many other obligations I have committed to, has been challenging, yet to live well, I have to balance all of life and ensure that I don't compromise my health.

Wellness is, by nature, a very broad topic. The Stinson Wellness Model is an attempt to identify major aspects of wellness in order to provide a workable framework with which to analyze our current wellness quotient and make decisions that lead to greater wellness.

It is important that the reader understand this book is not written with a solution in mind. Rather, it provides a process that will allow the reader to make decisions based on their personality and set of circumstances. Living well is the result of developing a personal way of knowing that is specific to each individual. As we come to know ourselves: our history, talents and passions, values and beliefs, and deep personal desires, we gain a sense of the person we are meant to be. We can then develop purpose and direction based on who we really are rather than what others want us to be. In the process we clarify our identity and begin to speak for ourselves - to find our personal voice in society.

This book reflects my own journey to understand how to live well. It is based on many years of listening to, learning from, and speaking with others who, whether friends or strangers, have shaped and influenced my thinking.

The focus of this book is to explain the structure of the Stinson Wellness Model and how it may be personally applied. I wrote it primarily for practitioners who have some background and understanding of the concept of wellness. As a result, the book is not a defense of the model (which will be found in journal articles). Instead, it was written informally to represent the spirit and organic nature of the model.

The Stinson Wellness Model is a framework that can be used to examine both group and personal wellness. Keep in mind that wellness is not simply an individual endeavor; personal wellness is intimately connected to the health of communities and groups of all sorts.

When a person is in crisis, they need to make immediate decisions that will help them survive. While in crisis, it is difficult to think long term and a person may need to take some drastic steps to get beyond the crisis stage. As a result, the Stinson Wellness Model is most helpful once a person regains a measure of stability. The model helps people build wellness back into their lives so that they can flourish.

I am indebted to many people for this model. First, my family and extended family have been a huge support. Without them I could never have completed this project. Second, many colleagues and friends have journeyed with me and given feedback and thoughtful insight. Lastly, I am grateful to many presenters, professors, and organizations for providing food for thought. In particular, I have benefited from over 25 years of work at Trinity Western University, where friends and activities constantly stimulate thoughts about wellness.

Aligning|Life

INTRODUCTION

During the 2011 British Open Championship, a television announcer described Darren Clarke, who was striding toward victory, as a great golfer and person: "He is every man's man. He smokes, enjoys a pint or two, and drives fast cars. ... Everyone likes him."

Winning the British Open was a significant achievement, and in that snapshot moment Clarke seemed to have everything going for him. Yet Clarke's journey included overcoming a major life blow when his wife died of cancer five years earlier. Fast forward to the 2011 British Open, as he putted out on the 18th green, his fiancé was in the crowd to cheer his victory. Clark had indeed risen to the challenges of life both personally and professionally.

Clarke is a celebrity I would enjoy meeting because he seems to be a normal person who lives authentically and in doing so lives well. But what does it mean to live well? Does it mean a person is successful at their vocation? Perhaps living well is about living a healthy life, or maybe it has to do with a positive outlook like the one that helped Clarke overcome the tragedy of his wife's illness and death. Although I do not know the details of Clark's private life and his wellness choices, there is something special about seeing personal and professional lives align well.

The Stinson Wellness Model is all about aligning life well. In writing this book, I am contending that living well is about how a person lives all of life, the good, the difficult, and everything in between. This book is an attempt to talk about how the average person can understand what it looks like for them to live well. It will also help personalize decision making so the reader can live a well-rounded and productive life.

Who are you? Who are you becoming?

Who are you? We rarely ask others this question, but it would help us get to know each other on a deeper level if we did. Instead we ask: *How* are you? *What* do you do for a living? What do you do in your spare time? If I asked you who you really are, what would you say? How do you define yourself? Is it by your vocation or family? Or is it by a passion such as an athletic sport or artistic endeavor? I am a skier ... I am a photographer ... Who are you down deep, where most people cannot see?

Who are you becoming? Who do you hope to be in a year? What about in five years? Have you dared to dream that far ahead? If you have, what system do you have in place that will help you become that person?

Notice I have not framed the questions around what you have achieved, or hope to achieve. Goals are often related to completing a task (something you want to do). I am not against goals and accomplishments, but *who* do you want to be in five years? In addition to the things we hope to achieve, we need to become intentional about the type of people we are becoming. Too often we focus on our "bucket list" of things we want to do and acquire, but neglect to nurture the growth of our character.

I work at a university and my colleagues and I recognize that the transition from school to work is a challenge that causes students to feel a lot of fear and uncertainty. At certain points in life, like graduation, questions about direction and becoming are extremely poignant. Despite the fact that students need direction at graduation, it is only one point in a lifelong journey of determining purpose and searching for meaning. *Who am I and who am I becoming?* Each day we live, we have the opportunity to alter who we are becoming by making small choices that move us in a chosen direction.

In this book, I am suggesting that the question, 'who am I and who am I becoming,' is very much connected with the question, 'how can we live life well?' Clearly these are very personal questions. Living well might then look quite different for me than it does you. Rightly so, because, even though we are all fundamentally human with many commonalities, we have different values, grew up in different cultures, and have different talents and passions. Living well has to do with living from the inside out, rather than being pulled by the cultural current of the day. This is what I see as aligned living - when the inside parallels the outside. To live well then, we must know who we are so that we can act with intentionality to move forward, in alignment. This involves decision making, another key aspect of wellness. The journey of living well requires us to discover who we are on the inside, something we can do only if we take the time to listen to our lives.

Listen to your life

Who are your heroes? What have they modeled that you would like to be true of your life? How would your life be different if you were living closer to your ideals than you are now?

In the back of all our minds are dreams, ideals, and expectations. When asked what it means to live well, we, to some extent, compare our realities with our ideals. The problem is that many of us dream but fail to develop strategies that will help us accomplish those dreams.

Parker Palmer (2000), in a book entitled *Let Your Life Speak*, challenges us to listen to guidance from within. He starts by explaining his approach to life when he was in his thirties:

> "So I lined up the loftiest ideals I could find and set out to achieve them. The results were rarely admirable, often laughable, and sometimes grotesque. But always they were unreal, a distortion of my true self – as must be the case when one lives from the outside in, not the inside out. I had simply found a "noble" way to live a life that was not my own, a life spent imitating heroes instead of listening to my heart" (p. 3).

He goes on to challenge us to listen to our hearts:

> "Before I can tell my life what I want to do with it, I must listen to my life telling me who I am. I must listen for the truths and values at the heart of my own identity, not the standards by which I must live – but the standards by which I cannot help but live if I am living my own life" (pp. 4-5).

In order to live well, we must look inside and live from the inside out.

SECTION ONE

FOUNDATIONS OF THE WELLNESS MODEL

CHAPTER ONE
Wellness: The Historical Context

The concept of wellness has deep historical roots and has changed over time. Aristotle defined good health in terms of moderation and limiting excess (Myers, 2008). The first written record of the English word "wellness" was in 1654 when a Scot, Lord Wariston, made an entry in his diary commenting that he was thankful for his daughter's "wealnesse" (Miller, 2005, p. 84). From the Middle Ages until the middle of the twentieth century, wellness was understood to be the antonym of illness (Miller, 2005). In other words, if a person was not sick, they were considered well. In the 1950s, wellness emerged in reference to active promotion of lifestyle changes that optimize a person's potential. By the 1970s, the wellness movement began to be popularized (Miller, 2005).

During the scientific revolution, Descartes and others differentiated between the body and the mind, which served to fragment a holistic interpretation of human functioning (Myers, 2008). It was not until the last half of the twentieth century that a tripartite perspective emerged to define the key components of humanity – body, mind, and spirit (Larson, 1999). These three components are often referenced today in wellness literature and were solidified when the World Health Organization (WHO) changed the definition of health, in 1958, from a medical model to a holistic interpretation. The World Health Organization defined health as "physical, mental, and social well-being, not merely the absence of disease" (1948, p. 1). This redefinition changed the concept from an either/or perspective to a continuum. Rather than a person being either sick or well, the new paradigm allowed for a continuum that extends from illness to average health at the midpoint and high-level wellness at the other extreme (Travis & Ryan, 1981, 1988, 2004).

In 1986 the first International Conference on Health Promotion was held in Ottawa, Canada. Discussions revolved around the actions to be taken with respect to "expectations for a new public health movement around the world" (World Health Organization, 1986). Health promotion, as understood in the Ottawa Charter, recognized that for people to live healthy lives, they needed to have increasing control over the means by which to improve their health.

"To reach a state of complete physical, mental and social well-being, an individual or group must be able to identify and to realize aspirations, to satisfy needs, and to change or cope with the environment. Health is, therefore, seen as a resource for everyday life, not the objective of living" (World Health Organization, 1986).

The charter also broadened the discussion from health issues and the health sector, to the responsibility of groups, particularly political entities that impact wellbeing through policy and resource allocation. They identified that the fundamental conditions and resources needed to achieve health are: "peace, shelter, education, food, income, a stable echo-system, sustainable resources, social justice and equity" (World Health Organization, 1986). The resulting implication of this Charter is that the responsibility for health and wellbeing relies on many segments of society. By working well together these groups will be able to provide an optimal environment in which people and groups are able to make positive choices that result in the opportunity to flourish.

Using a holistic perspective, the World Health Organization defines wellness in the following way:

[Wellness is] "… the optimal state of health of individuals and groups. There are two focal concerns: the realization of the fullest potential of an individual physically, psychologically, socially, spiritually and economically, and the fulfillment of one's role expectations in the family, community, place of worship, workplace and other settings" (Smith,

Tang, & Nutbeam, 2006, p. 5).

These World Health Organization definitions provide the foundational concepts for the development of current wellness theory.

Halbert Louis Dunn was a medical doctor and statistician who built on the changes initiated by the World Health Organization. His primary interests were related to the impact of infectious diseases on large groups of people, which caused many deaths globally. He believed that by living well, a society could reduce the spread of disease and possibly eliminate widespread impact of disease around the world (Miller, 2005). Dunn was frustrated with the medical profession's narrow biological perspective and emphasized both the mental and spiritual dimensions of wellness. In Dunn's view, Western culture took a fragmented approach by separating the body, the mind, and the spirit. He believed high-level wellness was directly related to harmony of the body, the mind, and the spirit (Miller, 2005). Dunn (1961) defined wellness as "an integrated method of functioning which is oriented toward maximizing the potential of which the individual is capable" (pp. 4-5). He created a health grid that helped diagram his understanding of wellness. It involved four quadrants: poor health, protected poor health, emergent high-level wellness, and high-level wellness (Miller, 2005). John Travis subsequently built on Dunn's work to create a wellness inventory involving twelve different dimensions based on a continuum, with premature death at one end point and high-level wellness at the other (Miller, 2005).

During the 1970's, the University of Wisconsin - Stevens Point created the first university wellness program after a nurse attended one of Travis's workshops. Bill Hettler, a university staff physician, stimulated by Travis' work, developed his own wellness inventory that was widely used on campuses across North America. He called it the Lifestyle Assessment Questionnaire. It is still in use, but is now marketed under the name Testwell. Hettler's model involves six dimensions of wellness: social, occupational, spiritual, physical, intellectual, and emotional (Hettler, 1998). One of Hettler's legacies is the National Wellness Institute, which began in 1977, and has been hosted every year at the Stevens Point campus. Hettler's work helped spread the wellness movement in the United States (Miller, 2005).

Donald Ardell is noted as being the person who popularized the term wellness, due in part to his engaging writing style. He expanded on the idea of high-level wellness from Dunn's work, has written many books, founded a wellness center, and has a thriving website, which includes a wellness newsletter entitled the Ardell Wellness Report (Miller, 2005). It is significant to understand that Ardell, Hettler, and others were contemporaries who influenced each other, even though they differed in their individual perspectives. Where Ardell is somewhat unique is that he has "pursued wellness from a rationalist and secular point of view," in contrast to others who viewed spirituality to be an important element of wellness (Hettler, 1998). At the 2004 National Wellness Conference, Ardell argued that the wellness movement would be better off without the concern for spiritual wellbeing (Miller, 2005).

Archer, Probert, and Gage (1987) defined wellness as "the process and state of a quest for maximum human functioning that involves the body, mind and spirit" (p. 311). Their definition represents a psychological perspective that is consistent with the psychodynamic and psychosocial theories represented by Jung (1933) and Maslow (1970), where "wellness may be viewed as an intrinsic motivation toward self-actualization and fulfillment" (Myers & Williard, 2003, pp. 145-146).

Jane Myers, whose background is in the counseling profession, is a prolific researcher on the topic of wellness. In 1992, Myers and Sweeney created a counseling-based wellness model entitled the Wheel of Wellness. The wellness assessment instrument that followed was named the Wellness Evaluation of Lifestyle (Myers, 2008). More recently, Myers et al. (2000) defined wellness as:

> "… a way of life oriented toward optimal health and well-being, in which body, mind, and spirit are integrated by the individual to live life more fully within the human and natural community. Ideally, it is the optimum state of health and well-being that each individual is capable of achieving" (Myers & Williard, 2003, p. 146).

In 1992, Myers argued that the counseling profession, as represented by the American Counseling Association, needed to move from a medical model to a preventative model involving optimal health and wellness. She proposed a resolution that called for: "… the counseling and development professions' position as advocate toward a goal of optimum health and wellness within our society" (p. 136).

In 2004, Hattie, Myers, and Sweeney analyzed a large amount of data collected with the Wellness Evaluation of Lifestyle and proposed a new model called the Indivisible Self: An Evidenced-Based Model of Wellness. Using structural equation modeling, they confirmed the seventeen components used in the Wheel of Wellness. After further investigation, the new model was developed. This new model, which is empirically based and "ecological," identifies four contexts that are integral to personal wellness: local (safety), institutional (policies and laws), global (world events) and chronometrical (lifespan) (Myers, 2008).

In Europe, the definition of wellness evolved quite differently in that they associate wellness with beauty, pleasure, and quality of life. The spa industry continues to play a significant role in defining wellness in European popular culture. The 'spa experience' represents the sentiment of Europeans who are comfortable with embracing the pleasure principle. As one study puts it: "Prosecco and Cappuccino were the insignia of a culturally refined 'wellness,' in which the cultural bourgeoisie proclaimed its hegemony: it was no longer the quantity of pleasure that counted, but its quality" (Horx, n.d., p. 7). Wellness has also become increasingly associated with beauty in general and in particular, the pursuit of a beautiful body (Illing, 1999, p. 8; Bingle, n.d., p. 6; Miller, 2005).

Another perspective that must be mentioned in this section is the field of positive psychology, in which wellbeing and human flourishing are central components of study. What makes a person happy and what mechanisms allow a person to flourish? This research plays a significant part in the discussion of wellness. Historically two juxtaposed philosophic perspectives have defined the study of wellbeing. The first philosophical position is that hedonia (hedonism) - personal enjoyment and feeling good - is the hallmark of living a satisfied and happy life. Eudaimonia, the second philosophical position, suggests that happiness results from living in congruence with one's true nature or daimon and actualizing a person's human potential (Deci & Ryan, 2006). *Feeling* good is more closely aligned with hedonia, while *doing* good is primarily associated with eudaimonia (Norrish, 2013). More recently researchers have recognized that hedonia and eudaimonia overlap and as a result the two philosophic perspectives are now being integrated. "The position taken by Waterman and colleagues is that, if a person experiences eudaimonic living he or she will necessarily also experience hedonic enjoyment; however not all hedonic enjoyment is derived from eudaimonic living" (Deci & Ryan, 2006, p. 3). Several theorists have identified structures that measure wellbeing, one of which is titled the Flourishing Scale, designed by Diener and colleagues (Diener et al, 2009). A focused discussion about the implications of this field of study is included in chapter two.

From 1950 to 1990, there was a relatively consistent understanding of the term wellness in North America, which involved promoting optimal health through lifestyle change. Since then, the meanings of the word have multiplied and mutated (Miller, 2005). Today, the use of the term wellness has become so diffused that it can refer to anything from a green laundry detergent, to a New Age healing clinic or a walk to promote awareness about obesity. Despite the variety of uses and definitions, I have chosen to use a more academic understanding of the term wellness, based on the definitions set out by the World Health Organization: definitions which represent a holistic view of life.

The concept of wellness is deeply rooted in several related terms, such as health, wellbeing, optimal living, and even pleasure. Definitions and theoretical models vary widely and involve several fields of study. Within this context, why would another type of wellness model be needed? The answer is that the Stinson Wellness Model approaches the concept of wellness from a very different perspective than most, although Dunn seem to share this view by referring to wellness as "maturity in wholeness" (1961, pp. 143-150). The Stinson Wellness Model helps people build wellness into their lives by encouraging wise decision making and authentic living in order for a person to contribute their unique talents and skills to the society in which they live.

CHAPTER TWO
Framing the Stinson Wellness Model

Chapter one provided a brief historical background related to wellness. This chapter is devoted to framing the conversation in practical terms. Like a good conversation, the chapter may take some unexpected turns because of the breadth of the topic, but these detours will be drawn together in the end to provide a framework within which the wellness model can be best understood.

Definitions

Since the term wellness has become so diffused in North American culture it is helpful to begin with definitions and then identify the implications associated with them.

The Stinson Wellness Model is based on the World Health Organization's (WHO) holistic definitions of health and wellbeing, which state that health is "more than the absence of disease," but is a "resource for everyday life" (WHO, The Ottawa Charter, 1986):

> "To reach a state of complete physical, mental and social well-being, an individual or group must be able to identify and to realize aspirations, to satisfy needs, and to change or cope with the environment ... [wellbeing] is created and lived by people within the settings of their everyday life; where they learn, work, play and love ..."

The World Health Organization definition of wellness is:

> "… the optimal state of health of individuals and groups. There are two focal concerns: the realization of the fullest potential of an individual physically, psychologically, socially, spiritually and economically, and the fulfillment of one's role expectations in the family, community, place of worship, workplace and other settings" (Smith, Tang, & Nutbeam, 2006, p. 5).

These definitions help us understand that while wellness includes physical health, wellness is the complete or whole state of a person's physical, mental, social, spiritual and economic wellbeing. There is a recognition that people that live well can identify and have found an optimal way of living that is better than other ways of living. An assumption is made that there are mechanisms available to people that allow them to have some control over elements of their lives and as a result they are able to realize their aspirations and satisfy their needs or change their environment. And finally, there is recognition that wellness includes personal fulfillment within a person's community. Wellness then, is holistic in nature and views each individual as a whole being living within the context of their community.

Wellbeing and Human Flourishing

The terms wellbeing and human flourishing are intimately linked to the discussion of wellness because they force us to define in greater detail what wellbeing and flourishing really is. Within ethical philosophy, the ultimate goal of living well has been understood to be personal happiness (Waterman et al, 2008). What constitutes happiness and the mechanisms that promote happiness align with two broad philosophical traditions; hedonism and eudaimonia (Deci & Ryan, 2008; Keyes & Annas, 2009; Ryff & Keys, 1995; Waterman et al, 2008).

Hedonia or headonsim as we know it, has to do with a person's subjective evaluation of his or her own happiness (Deci & Ryan, 2008). Those who experience higher levels of happiness are believed to have a greater sense of wellbeing. Hedonism focuses on personal pleasure and enjoyable experiences while minimizing pain (Norrish et al, 2013; Waterman et al, 2008).

The second philosophic stream is eudaimonia. "Where hedonic approaches focus on how people feel, eudiamonic approaches focus on what people do, how they act, and the choices they make" (Norrish et al, p. 148).

"Eudiamonistic ethics can be traced to the work of Aristotle (trans. 1985) and proposes that the goal of human functioning is to live in a manner consistent with one's daimon, or true self, where the daimon represents one's best potentials. "Living in truth to the daimon" entails selecting life goals on the basis of one's inherent nature, with the pursuit of such goals giving purpose and meaning to one's life" (Waterman et al, 2008, p. 42).

Living well from a eudaimonic perspective entails happiness that comes from self-acceptance, positive relations with others, personal growth, purpose in life and environmental mastery (Ryff & Singer, 2008).

Recently there has been increasing recognition that hedonia and eudiamonia are not juxtaposed but are, in fact, related (Keyes & Annas, 2009; Norrish et al, 2013). Keyes and Annas argue that experiences that are eudaimonistic are often pleasurable and that eudiamonic lifestyles are more about "the quality of your life as a whole, as opposed to just having good feelings, or getting what you want, or enjoying something you are doing" (2009, p. 198).

Simply put, when people feel good and are doing things that are aligned with what they believe and what they find meaningful or fulfilling, they are more likely to have higher levels of life satisfaction. The Stinson Wellness Model acknowledges both hedonia and eudiamonia by recognizing that meaning and fulfillment over a lifetime are facilitated by wise decision making that aligns with a person's core—their daimon. The model helps to operationalize many of the broad concepts that are foundational to wellbeing. By making wise decisions, a person is able to move, decision by decision, toward wellness allowing them to flourish in their own unique way.

Additional Implications

Some additional implications that flow from this way of thinking are that wellness is a life long journey and that rebalancing along the way is a given. When something of consequence happens in one part of a person's life, there are likely to be ripples in related spheres of life and adjustments will need to be made in multiple areas.

Another implication is that to live well, a person has to live authentically, acknowledging their talents and skills, strengths and weaknesses, passions and drives. Authenticity requires that people understand who they are and to live life from within, instead of being driven by external expectations. Wellness is intensely personal and cannot be defined simply by stages or steps but is concerned with a quality of life - one that suits each individual in their own unique way.

Finally, because personal wellness is interconnected with relationships and communities, living well has an impact on the people we live with on a day-to-day basis. And conversely, the interactions of others can have a profound impact on us. So we need to think carefully about how the interaction between individuals creates or detracts from building wellness into communities. Living well provides the foundation for giving back to a person's community in healthy and authentic ways. True wellness is not selfish, setting up boundaries that keep people and obligations out, but rather sets up boundaries so that a person can give to others in his or her community without becoming needy and sick in the process. Every individual has a responsibility to live well and to contribute positively to his or her society.

These implications are significant. How can a wellness model even begin to address them all? How can a model accommodate the individual nature of living well with the broader need to live well within community? The answer is twofold. First, the model needs to be personalized, allowing each individual to do their own soul searching to understand what wellness could look like for them as they live in their own unique community. Second, because what we do today impacts wellness tomorrow, it makes sense to focus on decision making that aligns with a person's ethos and identity as the means of moving toward wellness. The next section identifies the core of the Stinson Wellness Model.

The Wellness Equation

An assumption of the Wellness Model is that the alignment of interior and exterior lives results in authentic wellbeing. This means that intentional actions must flow out of self-knowledge. Decision-making in a topsy-turvy world becomes highly important to wellness! There is an almost mathematic elegance about it: the degree of Wellness equals circumstances multiplied by the sum of wise decision making and alignment.

$$\text{Wellness} = C (D + A)$$

"C" stands for Circumstances. Every individual lives within a set of circumstances. Some circumstances are beyond a person's control. Others are the result of intentional or unintentional decision making. Career paths may include both types of circumstances. For example, a person may make intentional choices about their education with a plan to work in a specific field, but along the way may encounter circumstances beyond their control that move them in a different direction. The economic crisis of 2008 impacted the careers of many people who did not make any conscious choices that caused the crisis. Regardless of circumstances, a person's journey toward wellness involves making wise decisions.

We often understand circumstances to be limiting factors to living life as we would wish—and to some extent they are—however in the Stinson Wellness model they are viewed as somewhat neutral. This is not because we never encounter negative circumstances, we all face these, but even in these challenging circumstances the solution is always to make wise decisions that help reduce the negative impact of the situation. We all know people who have overcome tremendous challenges and in so doing have become great examples of what it looks like to live well.

"D" refers to wise Decision Making, while "A" refers to Alignment. The frequency with which a person makes wise and aligned decisions has a multiplying effect on a person's wellness. Poor decisions have the same multiplying factor, but with negative results.

The Stinson Wellness Model provides a framework by which individuals can evaluate and align their decisions based on who they are internally and what they value or believe about life. In addition, the model recognizes that every person lives within their own unique context with ongoing circumstantial input. As Covey (2004) puts it:

"All of us can consciously decide to leave behind a life of mediocrity and to live a life of greatness - at home, at work and in the community. No matter what our circumstances may be, such a decision can be made by everyone of us - whether that greatness is manifest by choosing to have a magnificent spirit in facing an incurable disease, by simply making a difference in the life of a child, giving that child a sense of worth and potential, by becoming a change-catalyst inside an organization, or by becoming an initiator of a great cause in society. We all have the power to decide to live a great life, or even simpler, to have not only a good day, but a great day" (p. 29).

This may seem self-evident to many. Obviously if we make good decisions that fit for us, one would think that we would avoid many of the problems that seem to crop up on a daily basis. But it's not that simple. We have beliefs about circumstances and ourselves that may take us in the wrong direction without realizing it.

Mindset

Do you see circumstances as limiters or modifiers? Are circumstances a brick wall or a doorway? Are you stuck in a rut? Have you given up hope of changing your life? Carol S. Dweck, in a book entitled *Mindset: The New Psychology of Success*, makes the following statement:

"For twenty years, my research has shown that the view you adopt for yourself profoundly affects the way you lead your life. It can determine whether you become the person you want to be and whether you accomplish the things you value. ... Believing that your qualities are carved in stone – the fixed mindset – creates an urgency to prove yourself over and over. ... Every situation is evaluated: Will I succeed or fail? Will I look smart or dumb? Will I be accepted or rejected? Will I feel like a winner or a loser? ... The growth mindset is based on the belief that your basic qualities are things you can cultivate through your efforts. Although people may differ in every which way – in their talents and aptitudes, interests, or temperaments – everyone can change and grow through application and experience. ... The passion for stretching yourself and sticking to it, even (or especially) when it's not going well, is the hallmark of the growth mindset. This is the mindset that allows people to thrive during some of the most challenging times in their lives" (2007, pp. 6-7).

Throughout her book, Dweck provides many examples of how people who believe they can learn and grow are willing to take risks and develop a growth mindset.

In a study on voice and wellbeing among older adults in care settings, the older (and wiser) adults identified what often are externally perceived as barriers to wellbeing, such as hearing issues and system pressures, as modifiers rather than barriers (Richardson, 2010). It is all about persistence, adaptation, and 'work arounds,' they said. You can choose to open or shut a door, or access a window. Learning to see life challenges as opportunities for development and wise decision making allows people to embrace the concepts of the wellness model.

What do you believe about yourself? Do you have a fixed mindset or a growth mindset? Are you willing to risk carefully, to grow and change? Will you take the time to try and understand who you are and how that could be expressed authentically in your lifestyle? Are you willing to make small changes that move you in the direction you want to go? We all have the opportunity for personal transformation if we develop a growth mindset.

Intentionality: Strategic and Tactical Wellness

Who are you? Who are you becoming? These two questions suggest that who you are now can change as you journey into the future and that you have some control over how your future develops. If Dweck is right, we all have limitations and strengths, but the difference between those who succeed and those who do not is whether a person is willing to act on their beliefs to create positive change.

Change involves moving in a direction. We are all journeying through life and regardless of our perception on how long we have to live; we need to keep moving and growing. Along the way we will encounter limitations and roadblocks, some of which we do not control, but the goal is to overcome limitations and find a way around the roadblocks. Because life is an organic mix of the plans, hopes, and dreams, with challenges encountered along the way, our planning needs to be organic in nature - a mix of strategic and tactical planning.

Strategic planning is largely about envisioning where we want to go and then working out the steps to get there. This is a very important and helpful process but it involves being able to control many of the elements that allow the goal to be achieved.

Tactical planning has to do with being flexible enough to take advantage of opportunities that present themselves along the way. Where strategic planners develop a plan of action, the tactical planners anticipate opportunities and respond to them as they emerge.

Most people have a preference for one or the other. Those who like to have a plan in front of them gravitate toward strategic planning. Those who are more spontaneous and sensitive to their surroundings prefer to respond to opportunities.

The organic quality of living well requires a combination of the two. People need to dream about who they can become based on their talents and strengths. They need to set goals and move in their chosen directions. But they should also be aware of their surroundings and the opportunities that may come their way. By anticipating opportunities that fit their direction of travel and by preparing ahead of time, a person is able to make quick but wise decisions to engage opportunities before they are lost. Education is one form of preparation. For example, learning a computer program might be a very useful way to prepare. You never know when it may come in handy and it may actually allow you to move more quickly into a tactical opportunity.

What is your preference? What long and short term goals have you set for yourself? Do you have a clear direction of travel that will allow you to take opportunities that may come up? Are you willing to put some effort into preparing for possible opportunities?

Developing greater personal awareness, seeking to live authentically, dreaming about what could be in the future and being willing to make small but intentional changes are some of the critical dynamics that allow a person to fully engage the Stinson Wellness Model. Where are you at with this? Are you willing to engage the journey?

CHAPTER THREE
Description of the Stinson Wellness Model

The goal of the Stinson Wellness Model is to help you discover who you are so that you can live authentically from the inside out. The model is comprised of the 'layers of life' and four 'pillars of wellness.'

The layers of life help define key aspects of life which are all part of human existence but that have substantially different qualities. The graphical representation of the Stinson Wellness Model (figure 1) helps to visualize the model. In this chapter, I will define and present an overview of the layers of life and the pillars of wellness. In the next section of the book, we will explore each of the pillars more deeply.

Layers of Life

The layers of life sandwich the four pillars of wellness and are both influenced and influential to them. The smaller rectangles represent the individual while the larger rectangles represent a broader environmental context. Conceptually, the upper levels are the external aspects of our lives while the lower levels represent internal elements. In the graphic you will see that the large rectangle on the top entitled environment/community, contains the smaller rectangle entitled home/work, which is our immediate environmental context. Just below that layer is a rectangle entitled lifestyle. This is the external representation of who we are and where we interact with others in our environment. The four pillars of wellness, purpose, balance, congruence and sustainability link

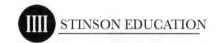

STINSON EDUCATION

STINSON WELLNESS MODEL

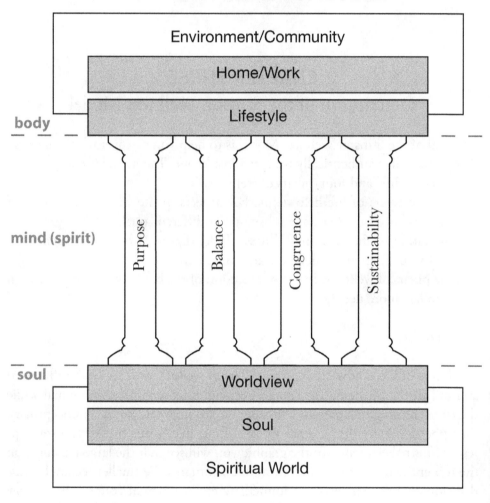

Figure 1

all of the layers of life, but are most clearly seen in the interaction between the worldview and lifestyle layers. Below the pillars is a similar construct to the upper layers, representing our internal lives. A rectangle entitled worldview, represents thinking patterns, emotions, identity and all the internal aspects of personhood. Below is a large rectangle representing the spiritual world. Within this rectangle is a smaller rectangle entitled, soul. The soul represents a person's personal identity within the spiritual world. Let's begin at the top of the diagram and work our way downward.

Environment and Community

The environment and community layer is the first external, topmost layer. Environment/community influence and are influenced by all other aspects of the model. We can think of environment and community on several levels of meaning.

At the broadest level, we are all a part of the cosmos. On a more concrete level, we are all global citizens. We share the world together. One obvious aspect of this layer is the environment. If one country pollutes or has a nuclear disaster, it has a worldwide impact. For some people, the impact may be catastrophic, while others may feel a minimal impact. The fact remains that we are all in this together and connected in many ways.

On another level, we are influenced by our place of origin. The laws and culture of a particular country influence who we are, how we live, and what we value, along with a host of other attributes. In addition, there are regional, state or provincial, and city differences that influence our lives. These are the broader environmental influences we encounter as we live life. As we delve further into the model, we will see how decision making influenced by the pillars, can affect even the broadest levels of the community and environment.

Home and Work

The immediate environment that we encounter every day has a tremendous influence on us. I have chosen to represent this layer with the words 'home' and 'work.' They are two primary aspects of life that involve a lot of time and significant relationships, and that have a major impact on personal wellbeing. We receive direct feedback from people in these environments who are important to us and as a result it is feedback that cannot be ignored.

Home, whatever that looks like for you, is a place that has a significant influence on your life. There are commonalities in being human, so on one hand we all share many drives and concerns. But the way we grew up, how we were treated, and the way we responded to challenges has shaped who we have become today. Because home is a critical part of the feedback loop in our environment, we need to be especially aware of the socialization and feedback associated with our personal family unit.

Work is another place where we are entwined with others in a way that is incredibly important. We get feedback such as annual performance reviews, promotions or demotions, raises or pay cuts, corner offices or cubicles, and high grades or failures. All of these things are a part of external feedback that speaks volumes about a person's performance to the recipient and those around them.

One of the reasons there are so many governmental organizations that regulate the workplace is the correlation between the job site and health and wellness. For example, the Canadian Centre for Occupational Health and Safety (CCOHS) states:

> "There is a strong connection between the health and well being of people and their work environments. When people feel valued, respected and satisfied in their jobs and work in safe, healthy environments, they are more likely to be more productive and committed to their work. Everyone can benefit from a healthy workplace" (2015).

Amabile and Kramer (2011) note "… that making headway on meaningful work brightens inner work life and boosts long-term performance. Real progress triggers positive emotions like satisfaction, gladness, even joy. It leads to a sense of accomplishment and self-worth as well as positive views of the work and, sometimes, the organization (p. 68)."

Your personality and the context you live in are unique to you. Families and family dynamics vary significantly. Work circumstances are also different from place to place. Whatever your world looks like, identify the people and places that have a strong and immediate influence on you and use the model to understand your situation. If needed, you can alter the model to fit your particular context. For example, home may look quite different from person to person. I spent most of my elementary and high school years in boarding schools and I often tell people that my classmates were my family. The school was home for much of the year. Similarly, work situations also vary. If you are a student, school is your workplace. Just because you do not get paid does not mean you are not working. Home may be the workplace of mothers who stay at home and take care of children. That is their work. So feel free to adapt the model so it fits your situation.

Lifestyle

The lifestyle layer consists of actions. It is the action outcome of our decisions or lack of decisions ... it is what we do. A person's lifestyle is the outward expression of their internal life. People see who we are through our lifestyles.

Lifestyle is where we interact with each other, and as a result it is also the place where we clash with others. We react to others primarily based on actions. But we all know that beneath actions are thought patterns. We try to interpret thought patterns through our observations of lifestyle behavior. Sometimes we can get angry with people because we interpret their actions to reflect negative attitudes that we think they hold. At times we may be correct, while at other times completely wrong. The point is that relationships are a two way street. We experience others and they experience us. When we share an experience we each interpret it in our own unique way in order to help understand it. Making meaning is very personal and people can share an experience yet come away from it with very different meanings.

Living closely with others means that we experience their actions on a regular basis. We begin to see patterns in their lifestyle and attitude more clearly. We see the good and the bad, the strengths and the weaknesses. And we are forced to deal with the reality that we are all flawed and at times are not very lovable. That is why our immediate environments (home and work) are so critical – these are the people who know us the best and see our flaws more clearly than we do. These are the people that can give us honest feedback, but they are also the people that can damage us the most if they do not have a healthy perspective on life.

Worldview

The worldview layer sits below the lifestyle layer and directs our actions. The concept of a worldview is large and complex. For the Stinson Wellness Model, the term worldview represents a person's internal world, complete with thought processes, emotions, perspectives, values, and beliefs. Given this framing of the term 'world view,' much of this layer is about patterns; how we view the world and our place in it at a very deep level of our heart and mind. Why is this layer so important? Much of moving toward wellness is connected to wise decision making. We make decisions all the time. Some decisions are very intentional and we have a good understanding of what we are doing. Others are, to a large extent, subconscious, and unless we spent time reflecting deeply, we can't always articulate our rationale for them. This is normal; we adopt patterns that allow us to make decisions quickly and automatically. What distinguishes this layer from others is that it is the internal, personal you or me in all its facets. We will delve into this aspect of the model and its importance a little later in Section Two when we discuss Worldview.

Spiritual World and Soul

Spirituality is another aspect of life where perspectives differ widely. The number of different belief systems in our world makes it challenging to create a model that has universal appeal. Some believe in a spiritual world, while others do not.

For those who do not believe in a spiritual world, this layer is ignored. But for those who do believe in a spiritual world, this layer provides a way to understand the connection between the physical world and the spiritual world. Because of the many different belief systems it will be up to each individual to figure out how their belief system fits the model.

The term 'soul' is used to identify a person's individual identity in the spiritual world. It refers to the personal aspect of spirituality within a broader spiritual context.

This is a section that many would say is of great importance and it should not be dismissed easily by saying, 'figure it out yourself.' If you feel this way, so do I. The fact, however, is that though I have given a lot of thought to this subject I'm no where near being able to write about it with any authority. It is a very interesting area that could use a lot of study. Where a person lands with some of these ideas will be intimately related to his or her personal belief system, so my encouragement is that as you seek to live life well that you begin to articulate your own personal beliefs on these matters.

Pillars of Wellness

The four pillars of wellness form a vertical connection between the upper and lower horizontal layers. The pillars are purpose, balance, congruence, and sustainability. The pillars of wellness are regularly revisited throughout life as people enter various life stages and encounter challenges that require them to re-evaluate how they are living.

The Purpose Pillar

Purpose has to do with who you are and your personal mission in life. Direction, closely related to purpose, refers to intentional movement toward a chosen outcome that matches your purpose. Obviously, people need self-awareness to discern their mission and goal in life, but for many this is a significant challenge that can easily trip them up and keep them from moving at all. Purpose is something developed over time as you travel through life and discover who you are, so often the best place to start is to begin moving in the direction that makes sense right now. Direction can change as purpose is gained.

Purpose is expressed differently depending on a person's personality. Obviously those who are driven set goals and work toward them, but easygoing people can also be intentional and work toward goals in a quiet but determined way. Implicit in the idea of wellness is a disciplined aspect to living that helps people make healthy and wise choices over decisions that are comfortable. Covey (2004) states:

> "I truly believe that discipline is the trait common to all successful people. I admire the work of insurance executive Albert E. N. Gray,

who spent a lifetime trying to discover the common denominator of success. Finally, he came to the simple but profound realization that although hard work, good luck and astute human relations are all important, the successful person has "formed the habit of doing things that failures don't like to do." Successful people don't like doing them either, necessarily. But their dislike is subordinated by the strength of their purpose" (p. 75).

Purpose provides the rationale and motivation to make and follow through on good choices that achieve wellness. Senge (1990) refers to this as personal mastery. "People with a high level of personal mastery share several basic characteristics. They have a special sense of purpose that lies behind their visions and goals. For such a person, a vision is a calling rather than simply a good idea "(p.142).

The Balance Pillar

The second pillar is balance. Balance is not simple or static. Occasionally, people find themselves off balance, so being one hundred percent balanced all of the time is an unrealistic goal. Becoming balanced and staying balanced requires regular adjustments to priorities and how time is spent.

Balance is also unique in that it feels right to the person on the balance beam! Someone may appear to be living a balanced life but may be radically out of step with where they need to be, and some may appear to be living chaotically but are actually living in overall balance. When life is fairly balanced, we are in control, feel good, and are able to manage the challenges we face. The key to living a balanced life is to be able to spot imbalance quickly and make small adjustments to compensate for the imbalance, rather than waiting to compensate and being forced to make a major adjustment to combat a crisis. Obviously some circumstances take us by surprise. But the better we are at understanding the patterns in our lives, the better we can be at anticipating imbalance.

Balance is related to purpose in that when we choose a direction that takes a lot of resources, we need to lean into our purpose in order to stay balanced. It is a little like balancing a bicycle or motorcycle. In order to stay balanced when a rider chooses to change direction, she needs to lean into the turn. Leaning too much or too little when rounding a corner will result in a crash. Balancing life in times of challenge can be equally as delicate, but with experience and constant adjustment great things can be accomplished without becoming too imbalanced and crashing.

While the concept of balance is easy to understand, those who live balanced lives have artfully developed methods and boundaries that protect them from the many pressures that can invade and disrupt a balanced lifestyle.

The Congruence Pillar

Congruence is the third pillar of wellness. Congruence means "the quality or state of agreeing or coinciding" (Woolf, 1980, p. 236). People who live well have found a relative state of congruence in critical areas of life. There is congruence between their beliefs and actions. Their understanding of who they are – their distinctiveness, passions, strengths, and weaknesses – coincide with their purpose in life and are firmly based on their personal worldview. Rogers (1961) suggested that congruence is the peak of personhood. A congruent person achieves an accurate "matching of experience, awareness and communication" (p. 339). Chickering (1990) adds that, "When fully realized, integrity is reflected in consistency of belief and behavior, of word and deed. Internal argument is minimal. … Achieving congruence is a lifelong task" (pp. 139-142).

Strong congruence relates to a mature sense of identity and authenticity, because a person's lifestyle matches their values and beliefs. They know who they are and have a clear sense of how they intend to live. Living in congruence is characterized by inner peace – even in the midst of complex and challenging environments.

The Sustainability Pillar

Lives that are lived well are sustainable. Everyone experiences being stretched and overwhelmed from time to time. This is natural. If, however, life becomes characterized by being overwhelmingly busy and stressed, we will likely encounter sickness of one sort or another. Sustainability is about pacing ourselves over time.

Life is far more sustainable when we are able to live well internally and externally within our environments. Consequently, greater sustainability is found when we live congruent lives. Acknowledging and using our strengths rather than operating within our weaknesses creates greater sustainability. To do this, a person has to say "no" to some good things in order to choose the best.

Sustainability has to do with managing the energy drain that is expended in multiple areas of life with the need to rejuvenate and re-energize. Both are important to living long and productive lives.

Wise Decision Making and Alignment

Each of the pillars has a question associated with it, which, if used in the decision-making process will lead to wiser decisions that align with a person's values and beliefs. This is how 'living from the inside out' is achieved. Below are the questions for each pillar:

> *Purpose: Does this take you in the direction you want to go?*
> *Balance: Are you taking a balanced approach?*
> *Congruence: Do your actions reflect your values and beliefs?*
> *Sustainability: Can you do this long term?*

In the process of answering these questions, a person has to look deeply into their values and beliefs to determine what type of decision authentically reflects who they are. By frequently making wise decisions, a person will move toward personal wellness.

Citizenship: Footprint in Society

We are all part of a society. Consequently every person has a footprint in his or her community. What kind of a footprint do you have? Do you take more than you give back to your community? Or do you give back more than you receive? Each of us needs to understand that we are participants in our communities. Giving to and receiving from others creates strength and unity within a society.

The challenge for people who live well is to contribute to others based on the gifts and skills they have to offer. It is a call to live authentically and to participate constructively in our communities. If we simply concentrate on what is good for us as individuals, we neglect our responsibilities to create healthy and sustainable communities. A significant aspect of wellness is being a productive citizen.

Aligning|Life

SECTION TWO

WORKING WITH THE WELLNESS MODEL

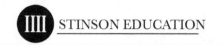

STINSON EDUCATION

STINSON WELLNESS MODEL

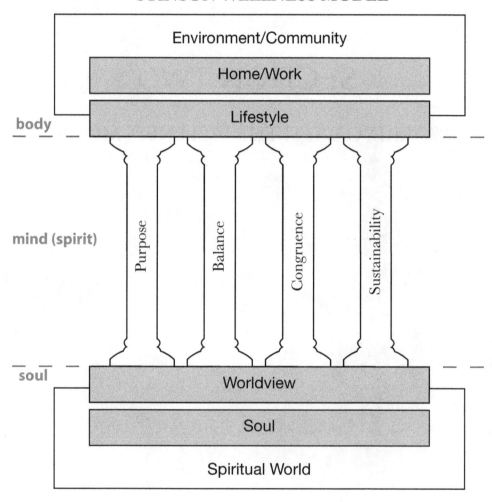

Figure 1

DISCUSSION ONE
The Art of Living Well

There is a strong temptation to try to create a formula or blueprint that people can use to live well. However, the reality is that because of the great variety of personalities, circumstances, values, and beliefs that make up peoples' lives, the process of living well is much more like an art form than a blueprint. In the last section, I described the Stinson Wellness Model. The remaining chapters are discussions of key issues related to the model, and particularly to the four pillars of wellness. Each reader will need to consider the implications and develop strategies that fit their personality and context. How will you do this? By acquiring the information, formulating an understanding of who you are, and living this knowledge out in wisdom.

Information, understanding, and wisdom

A lot of people think being educated has to do with learning information. This first level of learning is characterized by memorizing facts and other types of information long enough to regurgitate them on a test or use them in a conversation. This is a lower level of learning that is often quickly forgotten.

A second level of learning is when a person asks why and how? I call this understanding, because people not only have a good grasp of information, but also how it is used. A person who has understanding comprehends processes and is able to apply ideas in meaningful ways.

A third level of learning is wisdom. Those who are wise have a broad range of information at their fingertips, understand how things work, and have applied that understanding in their lives. Ultimately, those who live well have a level of wisdom they apply to their lives, resulting in benefits to those around them.

This is important because the art of living well fits into the wisdom category. People who live well have a sense of identity and live life with depth and consistency. As we discuss various aspects of wellness, recognize that living well is something that is learned and practiced over a lifetime.

Transformational Learning

If living well has to do with developing wisdom, how is this done? Is there a process that helps turn regular information and experiences into something that becomes meaningful and transformational in a person's life? Is this something we can actually control, or is wisdom gained passively as we live life?

When talking about wisdom, all sorts of values, religious beliefs, philosophical perspectives and cultural backgrounds come into play, so it is scary to give advice on how to find wisdom, however I am comfortable in explaining what has been helpful to me in terms of learning what I consider to be day-to-day wisdom.

About twenty years ago I began to wonder what transformational learning might look like? As an educator I hoped that what I was teaching would actually have a positive impact on others, so it was natural to wonder about how this might be done. In the process I reflected on things that have transformed my life and how I discovered them. The end result is a model that I called the Stinson Transformational Learning Model. In thinking about wellness both individually and collectively, I keep coming back to the model because I think it informs how meaningful learning happens. Think about your life. How have you learned who you are and what is important to you? How did you learn these things? I hope that a discussion of the transformational learning model will trigger some of your own thinking and enable you to be more intentional as you seek to live well.

We are all learners. What we choose to learn and how we prefer to learn differs from person to person. However, I believe that there are three active ingredients to transformational learning. Let me describe them first and then explain how they work together.

The first is what I call Information and which typically is second hand knowledge. Second hand knowledge is information that we have not experienced personally. What is taught in the classroom often falls into this category since it is information that someone else has developed, researched, theorized about or experienced. An example of this kind of knowledge would be the information that one could gain about how to fly an airplane by reading books or watching videos. A person may know a lot about flying an airplane but still never have flown one.

Recently, a friend named Tim who trains pilots for a major airline invited me to fly in a flight simulator with him. I came away with a huge respect and great thankfulness for the training pilots receive. One thing that struck me that day was that before a pilot gets to fly in the main flight simulator they train on more basic platforms. The first station is a wooden replica of the cockpit instruments. At this station, pilots train their brain and muscle memory so that they know where each function is located. When they have mastered that station, they move on to a smaller, computer based simulator to continue their training. Only after mastering those two stations do they move on to the main flight simulator.

The second observation is that this progression provides pilots with a transition from knowing about flying (second hand information) to experiencing the process of flying an airplane. Experiencing something is powerful. Prior to experiencing the simulator, I had played computer video games that allowed me to fly and I wondered how different they would be. The flight simulator was very different.

Walking up to a flight simulator, you see a cabin size room on legs but once inside it looks like the cockpit of an airplane--because it is a fully functioning cockpit. As Tim powered up the simulator, the windscreen came alive and it was as though we were looking down a runway outside. After Tim took off, he turned right and left to show us how realistic the graphics were. He made another sharp turn and asked us to look back out the door we came in, which he had intentionally left open. Though my stomach had reacted a little to the sharp turns, when I looked back it was clear that my queasiness was related to the visual graphics of the windscreen rather than motion because the simulator had not moved at all. Then he turned on the movement function, did some sharp turns and I almost threw up. At that point I really experienced the simulator.

Later, Tim let me 'land' the airplane. All I had to do was steer it onto the runway. Tim took care of the speed, the flaps and the rest of the things that needed to be done. Though I landed, the landing was very rough and I almost went off the runway trying to stop. I'm certain that just before landing Tim helped me correct so I would not crash.

The point of this story is that my experience in the simulator was powerful. I gained a far deeper appreciation for pilots and their expertise through the experience than if I had just read a story about how pilots fly airplanes. It also triggered thoughts about how and why things are set up the way they are in a cockpit and as I've already mentioned the experience caused me to reflect on the complexity of the skills that pilots learn in order to keep us safe in the air.

Remember, my experience was to land in a simulator with a great deal of help from a friend and with no risk to life and limb. I never left the ground. I experienced a simulation--which is helpful--but it's not the same as the real thing. Commercial pilots have years of flying experience. I'm glad they fly the airplanes rather than someone who has only flown a simulator.

The second active ingredient to transformational learning is our own personal experience. We learn things as we experience them (first hand experience). Because experiences are powerful they often trump theories that come in the form of second hand information. Everyone brings a different set of experiences to the learning process, which can result in similar experiences having different effects.

The third active ingredient is personal reflection. Without taking time to reflect, a person can have an experience but miss the meaning. Reflection is not just an idyllic, peaceful state of mind where all incongruities are avoided, but rather reflection is often characterized by mental wrestling. Reflection is done in many ways, using various techniques, but always with the same goal; to find congruity and meaning between experience and knowledge around us.

The transformational learning model is graphically represented in Figure 2.

Stinson Wellness Model

TRANSFORMATIONAL LEARNING MODEL

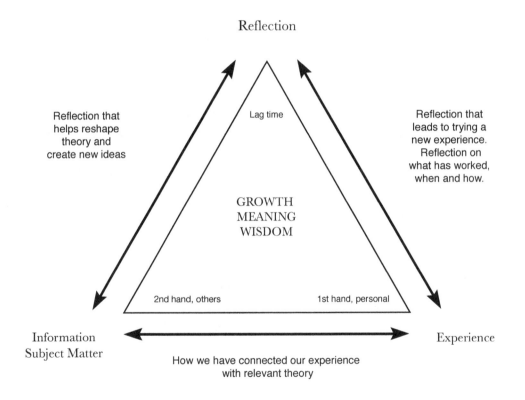

Reflection

Reflection that helps reshape theory and create new ideas

Lag time

Reflection that leads to trying a new experience. Reflection on what has worked, when and how.

GROWTH MEANING WISDOM

2nd hand, others

1st hand, personal

Information Subject Matter

Experience

How we have connected our experience with relevant theory

Figure 2

How does it work?

Transformational learning is intensely personal. When we bring our experience into the equation and look for meaning we personalize learning. Growth, meaning and wisdom are byproducts of mixing the three ingredients.

It does not really matter where the process begins. In the classroom it generally begins with new ideas from a lecture or readings. Often it involves understanding theories that others have developed. Teachers then use discussion or case studies to help link theories to concrete experience and to help us reflect on the meaning or application of the theory.

Flying the simulator was an experience that triggered reflection. At other points learning may begin with reflection - realizing something new based on an observation that was noteworthy.

Ultimately, the result of mixing these three ingredients is transformational learning. It is learning that changes and transforms our lives. It connects the head with the heart and hands. Transformational learning initiates action that is aligned with who we really are.

It is interesting to me that often common sense is linked with living well. The problem is that it is really 'uncommon sense' since so few people seem to have it. I suspect that if more of us were intentional about transformational learning and were more aware of the world around us that greater common sense would be developed.

As we dive deeper into the wellness model, it is important that we practice using a learning process that can help us grow and develop meaning in our lives. The transformational learning model provides this. It is another mechanism that can assist us with aligning our lives. My experience has been that all too often I have responded to the expectations of others rather than developing my own way of being and my own voice. I listened to external voices, not my own and as a result had a very hard time determining priorities. As I have developed my internal self, thought through who I am and what living well looks like for me, I have been able to live with greater vitality and purpose.

What type of learning is typically reflected in your life? What is the least used ingredient? Can you identify how you prefer to learn based on this model? How can you use the learning model to discover your true self? What does the art of living well look like for you?

DISCUSSION TWO: PURPOSE
Does This Take You in the Direction You Want to Go?

"Go confidently in the direction of your dreams. Live the life you have imagined."
Henry David Thoreau

What is your purpose in life? What are your dreams? Do you have a clearly defined direction of travel? "Following a deeper call in our lives means that something (an aim, a passion, an interest, a problem, an idea) attracts us enough to move us to action on its behalf and is important enough so that focusing on it directs our activities and provides our lives with a sense of meaning" (Leider, 1997, p. 33). Purpose is a very broad subject, which ranges from identifying a personal mission or calling in life to setting and achieving day-to-day goals that help us to live well within the context of that calling.

In the Stinson Wellness Model, purpose and congruence are connected; balance and sustainability are also connected. To find real purpose, a person must identify their true self or daimon as noted in the wellbeing literature. This concept is discussed further in the chapter on congruence, but it is important to note that as we develop a sense of our true selves, we adapt our purpose to fit who we are. We begin to think differently and alter our lifestyles appropriately. The lens of our worldview is altered to bring clarity to our identity, value and place in society. All of these elements are linked together and as we grow and learn, we mature, are able to live more consistently and strengthen our identity.

Purpose grows and is strengthened over time as we live intentionally. The starting point, however is to set some small goals and begin moving in the direction that makes the most sense right now. That is why this section is primarily about goals and goal setting.

We will begin by identifying three levels of purpose and end with goal setting because the way forward into greater wellness is by making small daily decisions that align with the larger mission or calling we have identified for our lives.

Levels of purpose

The concept of purpose seems to reference three different levels, all of which are important. The first is what I think of as the existential level. It is the broadest type of purpose and involves the deep questions of life. Why do I exist? What is my purpose on earth? A mix of concepts garnered from religion, philosophy, and science typically answers these questions – and each person has to find answers for themselves.

A second level deals with long-term goals related to aspects of life like career, education, or family commitments. These are goals that take years to accomplish and involve many practical considerations. Accomplishment of these goals is dependent on developing a sequence of short term goals that move a person closer and closer to their goal.

Existential beliefs frame how we live, so there is a connection between the first two levels if a person is living an aligned life. It takes a lot of work to synchronize the two layers, so it is common that the relationship between the two is not very clear.

A third level has to do with day-to-day living. The decisions we make each day should synchronize with short-term goals. The short-term goals should move us in the direction of accomplishing our long-term goals. At the same time, we need to live out our values and beliefs, which are often attached to existential goals. This is a challenging task and we often feel disjointed as we struggle to connect our day-to-day decisions with our goals and values.

Living well is a significant challenge. The process of making wise decisions that align with who we are helps us to live with purpose. So where do we go from here? How do we move forward?

Simply put, we need to understand the complexities of purpose, but then use simple, everyday techniques that help keep us on track. The fact is that change happens in the present, and small changes over time can move us a long way in the direction we want to go. So the goal is to live every day intentionally and with purpose.

Goals

People tend to drift without goals and direction, so it is important to articulate hopes and dreams. Some people have clearly defined goals and have developed strategies that help them accomplish their goals. If you are one of these people, you may want to skim this section. If you are a person who has struggled with setting goals and finding strategies that actually work for you, then hopefully this next section will be helpful.

Why do some of us struggle with goal setting and creating workable strategies? Many people do not set goals because they were never able to accomplish them in the past. I used to be one of those people. As I learned more about myself I changed several things that have helped me to live more intentionally.

The first change was based on the observation that my goals often failed because accomplishing them was tied to other people or things I did not control. One expert explained that goals you do not have direct control over need to be held on to lightly because you can only control your part of the goal. Now I set goals that focus primarily on what I control.

The second way I have changed my goal-setting practice is to think of a goal as a direction of travel. Now I think of goals as segments of travel toward a destination point. This helps me because I don't have to create large goals that have all the details figured out. I focus on taking one small step that takes me closer to the goal. At times I don't know what the step after that is--often because it involves something that I don't control. But by taking one step forward it opens doors and opportunities to move forward that were not available to me before.

There are many ways to get from point A to point B. Let me explain by using a travel analogy. If two different people planned a road trip across North America, from Seattle to New York, the routes could be quite different. One person could choose to take the fastest and largest highways across the continent to get to his destination, New York, as quickly as possible. If speed is the goal, then this might be an appropriate way for him to travel. A different person may plan a trip that takes her through as many out-of-the-way places as possible or to places that are on her bucket list. In planning the trip, each person makes choices about where and how they want to travel. Based on some of these choices, they then have to break the trip into segments with destinations and time frames.

Goal setting in life has similar characteristics. Most of the people who taught me goal-setting techniques seemed to be the people who were going from point A to point B as fast as possible. In a nutshell, I am not like them. I have found that very few things in life that are worthwhile are done quickly. By recognizing there are many ways to accomplish a goal and adopting a philosophy that life is not a race, I have been able to set a direction and work at my own speed to get there. When I run into a roadblock along the way, I adjust my direction, go around it, and get there eventually. Allowing for more organic goal setting and the ability to make adjustments along the way has helped me to set goals while living authentically and intentionally.

A final problem I continually ran into was discouragement. It seemed as though I could never accomplish my goals. I realized the problem was that I was setting goals that were too large. When I did not accomplish a goal, I got discouraged and quit. Discouragement led to procrastination. At that point I would not even start working on a goal because I already felt defeated. To deal with this I have learned to set small goals. If a goal seems too large and I see myself procrastinating, I ask, "What can I accomplish easily?" Then I change my goal to something I know I can accomplish and set out to do so. This technique is the secret to overcoming procrastination - breaking large goals into smaller, more manageable goals. The idea of moving toward a destination using steps that are easy for me to take has allowed me to accomplish far more and to pursue goals with greater determination.

With this discussion in mind, begin to dream. What are your hopes and dreams? Who would you like to become? What would you like to accomplish? What steps would help move you in that direction? Here are some guidelines for moving forward.

Begin by actually writing down your hopes and dreams. Some may be long term, bucket list items while others may already be in process and have an end in sight. Second, see if any of them can be grouped together. Often our goals cluster around our passions. By identifying the relationships between goals, we can usually work toward several of them at the same time. A third consideration is sequence. Will one goal provide the foundation for moving forward to the next?

It is not unlike planning the road trip from Seattle to New York. The primary goal is already identified. Now it is a matter of breaking the trip into sections based on a variety of considerations. Is there a dream destination along the way? Which friends would you like to visit? What are the roads like? What time frames need to be considered? One section of the travel plan needs to synchronize with the next until you get to New York.

The problem with this type of planning is that there are always unexpected circumstances that may cause you to adjust your plans. There could be road closures or vehicle accidents that complicate travel. In fact, you could be injured in an accident. If that happened, your trip could change completely. We cannot predict the future so we need to hold on to our plans lightly.

On a brighter note, opportunities to explore may also show up. One of the fun things about travel is that you meet people along the way who add to the richness of the journey. Spending time with them or allowing them to show you places you did not know about can be extremely rewarding. In the same way, we ought to treat life like a journey and be open to the opportunities that present themselves along the way. In the end, we may significantly alter our direction of travel or even change our ultimate destination.

In an earlier section, I explained strategic and tactical wellness. I believe the same principles apply to developing purpose. On one hand, we need to have a general sense of where we would like to go – a direction in life. On the other, we ought to live tactically by being aware of the opportunities that come our way and be able to makes choices quickly enough to take advantage of them. Both strategic and tactical planning should be applied to developing purpose.

Does this take me in the direction I want to go?

This question, if used regularly, helps keep us on course. It also forces us to look regularly at alignment. Do the day-to-day decisions I am making fit with my larger purpose? Am I moving forward in a way that reflects my values and beliefs?

Identifying purpose pushes individuals to look deep within. A friend of mine is a nurse and she often says, "Once a nurse, always a nurse." Her point is that she was trained to look for certain things as a nurse. Over time, these traits have become so en-grained in her that she cannot help but think like a nurse. Nursing is one of her passions. It is woven deeply into her lifestyle and worldview. Nursing also has a deep spiritual meaning for her. This alignment is powerful. Aligning purpose at all levels is what allows people to live with conviction and passion.

I am including a worksheet on goal setting that may be helpful for individuals who are not as comfortable with setting short-term goals. I have also included an explanation that will help the reader understand why each step is important.

Explanation of the Goal-Setting Worksheet

Each goal you set should be specific and have a time frame attached. Be realistic about how much you can accomplish. If you have a big goal, break it down into small, manageable pieces and develop a strategy that will help you accomplish it. One of my big goals is to make a trip to Africa. An example of a smaller goal to help me get to Africa is to research the cost and develop an itinerary. Once I have the cost, I can develop a savings strategy to pay for it. I will also need sub-goals that relate to other logistical issues such as: When do I need to get vaccinations and visas for the trip? Are there people I would like to visit on my trip? What do I need to communicate to them before leaving?

If your goal is bigger than one month, begin to break it down. What do you need to do each month if your goal will take a year? What do you need to do every six months to achieve a five-year goal? The key to successful goal setting is to break goals into small, easy-to-accomplish sub-goals that move you one step closer to accomplishing a large goal.

I want to do this because …

If a goal is someone else's idea, you may not have the motivation to achieve it. You have to choose your goals and value them. If you choose to set a goal, write

Stinson Wellness Model

GOAL SETTING WORKSHEET

In the next: _____ (timeframe)

I would like to: _____

I want to do this because ...

Barriers or obstacles I will encounter are ...

Resources/knowledge I need in order to do this are ...

I will get these resources/knowledge by ...

Figure 3

Sequential plan of action:

Note: Your sequential plan of action should help you overcome barriersand obstacles.

1.

2.

3.

4.

5.

6.

7.

8.

9.

10.

I will have accomplished my goal when ...

Figure 3

down your reasons why you are choosing to set the goal.

Barriers and obstacles I will encounter are …

Few people anticipate the obstacles they will encounter when they set a goal. Often these obstacles are easy to identify because we have encountered them before - in fact we have probably seen them multiple times before. They have likely been the reason for not achieving other goals. For example, if money is tight, the cost associated with a goal will be a problem to overcome. The reason I have not already gone to Africa is that I have never had enough extra money I could put toward this expensive trip. In addition, saving for the trip has to take priority over other things in life and frankly, the trip has often been a lower priority to other more important items. The point is that if I had unlimited time and money, I would have already accomplished my goal. Until I address the financial obstacle, I will not get to Africa. So identifying obstacles and designing a plan to overcome them is a critical aspect of succeeding at goal setting. These strategies then become a part of the plan of action.

Resources/knowledge I need in order to do this are …

Not having the knowledge and support needed to accomplish a goal can contribute to failure. As a result, we need to think about whether we have the resources needed to accomplish the goal. When it came to renovating my house, I had to hire an engineer to give me direction so that moving a support beam would not result in the house falling down. Good friends guided the design and construction of the project. An excellent framer did the framing and a great finish carpenter installed the kitchen cabinets. I was most successful as the person who cleaned up. There were many things I could not do, and I either had to hire help or learn how to do them myself.

It is important to identify the knowledge and resources you have at your disposal and the ones that you lack. What is needed for you to be successful? Make a list of these things.

Sequential plan of action ...

A plan of action identifies the order of steps you will take to accomplish your goal. The steps need to be sequential. Some things will have to be done before you can tackle other aspects of your goal. When renovating my house, I needed to draw plans and get building permits before starting. Once these were in place we could begin the construction phase. Similarly, it is important to set up a plan of action that is sequential and has strategies embedded in it that will help you overcome the obstacles you will encounter.

I will have accomplished my goal when ...

It is important to have a way of measuring when you have achieved your goal. These indicators should be very specific in nature. You should also have the flexibility to adjust your goals if needed by extending the deadline or reducing the amount you hope to get done if you encounter challenges. The key here is to recognize that any gain is a good gain. I used to have a boss who said when golfing, "If I am closer to the hole than before, it is a good shot." Usually we get discouraged when we do not meet our goals. Rather than being discouraged, we should view any movement forward as success. Be patient. We often set unrealistic goals without realizing it, so give yourself a break and celebrate forward movement. Adjust your goal and keep working.

DISCUSSION THREE: BALANCE
Are You Taking a Balanced Approach?

The image of a diamond helps explain the complexity of being human. Diamonds do not come out of the ground the way we see them in a ring. It is the process of grinding many facets in patterns, which reflect light that makes a diamond beautiful. Every well-cut diamond shimmers and shines when all the facets work together to collect the light and reflect it back with glittering brilliance.

Balance is like a diamond since there are many facets to our lives that need to work in sync for us to live well. There is an art to determining how much time and effort a person should exert on each facet. Balancing life is a very delicate and complicated endeavor.

Neglect

Have you ever taught someone how to ride a bike? How did you describe balance? What does balance feel like? How is it achieved? Balance in life is extremely difficult to describe because life feels good when we experience balance. It is only when life no longer feels good, that we are tipped off to the fact that we are experiencing imbalance. The realization occurs that we may need to make changes before we hit the ground! It is easier to begin a discussion about balance by discussing the lack of it - imbalance.

Good mountain bike riders are able to stay balanced in precarious positions. Part of what makes them exceptional is that they anticipate the impact of roots and rocks that will throw them off balance and adjust their riding accordingly to maintain their balance. So it is with life. To the extent that we recognize events that will throw us off balance and make appropriate corrections with strategic timing, we can live much more balanced lives. This ability to anticipate challenges and adjust for them in a timely fashion is a hallmark of living well.

Imbalance is often associated with neglect. Neglecting important aspects of life over a long period of time can lead to crisis situations. For example, if a person neglects their finances, they will soon get letters from creditors reminding them they have not yet paid their bills. If they fail to address this neglect, they will encounter severe consequences. This same pattern applies to people who ignore health considerations. If serious concerns are not addressed, a life crisis will likely be the result.

Much of life follows this pattern. If we completely neglect balance for lengthy periods of time, the consequences become severe. The goal of moving toward wellness is to ensure that we make balancing adjustments long before we find ourselves in crisis situations.

Person Specific

Balance is person specific. What might be balanced living for one may not be appropriate for another. I stay reasonably fit for a middle-aged guy who has an office job. But would my exercise routine work for a high-level athlete? Never. It would be neglectful for an athlete to use my exercise routine. The point is that balance, to some degree, is related to purpose. My purpose is different from a competitive athlete, so it is appropriate that my exercise level be different. Balance is an individual matter.

This brings us to another observation. We tend to like to operate in our areas of strength. This happens at the gym as well as in other areas of life. A person may exercise parts of their body that are the most fit rather than working on parts that need development. Or a person who is a good verbal communicator may prefer to talk more than working on writing skills that may not be as well developed. The application here is that we need to identify areas of neglect – usually things we do not enjoy – because that is where the greatest risk is located. We cannot let our weaknesses dominate our lives to the point that they undermine our strengths and abilities. Do your weaknesses dominate your strengths? This is another way to identify imbalance.

We all live with some imbalance in our lives. Living well seems to be more about managing small imbalances and remaining mostly balanced, rather than finding the perfect balance in all aspects of life, all of the time.

Imbalance can be identified in at least two ways. When we neglect an important part of life and life no longer feels right, we know we are imbalanced. The second indicator is when our weaknesses dominate our day-to-day experiences and we are no longer purpose focused.

Balance is related to Purpose

If we have a purpose for living, we ought to spend energy engaging that purpose. Living well always involves expending energy. It makes sense that we put energy into what we have chosen to do and who we are hoping to become. Spending energy in meaningful ways and being replenished by things that bring us joy add vitality and meaning to life.

As a young person, I got the impression that the primary goal in life was to pack my days as full as possible with things of value. I also thought I could run at one hundred percent all day, every day. I have since come to realize that balance is about both work and rest, choosing the best over what is good, and expending energy on things I value while being intentional about replenishing the energy I expend.

Balance on a bicycle is not necessarily about staying perpendicular to the road. Some people treat balance as though it is a static state of existence or a formula that helps a person stay at ninety degrees to the road for long periods of time. Balance in life, like balance on a bike, is accomplished by making many small adjustments that keep us upright. And, like the roads we bike on, our lives are not always straight and easy to navigate. We regularly have to change directions and lean into corners in order to stay balanced. Balancing life is an ongoing process of staying balanced as we lean into turns and avoid rocks and roots we encounter along the way.

Living well requires that we lean into our purpose. Things that are worthwhile normally take a great deal of time and energy. At times, managing purpose and balance well, actually moves us into a razor's edge type of living. We have to be very careful to lean into our purpose in a very exact way or we will end up crashing and getting hurt.

Speed is also a factor in successfully navigating balance. If we enter a corner too quickly, the amount of lean no longer matters because a crash is certain. Taking a corner too fast is never a good idea. The life application is that unrealistic time frames will normally result in a crash. Consequently, we need to be very aware of the speed at which we are traveling. The art of balance requires leaning into our purposes intentionally and carefully.

Balancing Time Commitments

Living well involves balancing multiple aspects of life, many of which seem to have a high-priority status. A few years ago, a friend created a seminar en-titled *Dropping Balls Gracefully*. His perspective was that many of us regularly commit more time than is realistic to any number of good causes. We accept commitments with the understanding that a certain amount of work is expect-ed of us. Over time, though, these commitments seem to expand and change beyond the original expectation and we find ourselves being stretched beyond our capacities. At this point the balls in the air that we have been juggling get out of control and begin to fall to the ground. My friend's seminar addressed the issue of what to do when we get too busy.

Note that this is not always someone else's fault. It is very common for people who want to do a good job to do more than was originally asked. As a result, the bar is raised and soon it becomes very difficult to "drop a ball" with the new expectations that have been put in place. That is why some people use the saying, "No good deed goes unpunished." What began as a good deed - going beyond what was required - turned into an onerous expectation. Usually we can temporarily manage the imbalance by becoming more efficient, but it is not uncommon for commitments to get out of control. Sometime before a crisis hits, a person needs to recognize that life is becoming imbalanced and find ways to drop balls gracefully to reduce their commitment level.

Conflicting Values and Priorities

Because balance has to do with all aspects of life, we often encounter conflict-ing values and priorities. You already know I would like to take a trip to Africa. It is a worthy and good goal. But since I have a family, achieving balance involves consideration for everyone, not just myself. By clarifying our family priorities we have been able to determine that going to Africa is not the highest priority. When priorities are not clearly defined we end up with conflicting priorities, which are often major obstacles to creating and maintaining balance.

Usually it is not a case of one value being good and the other bad. Often it is a competition between two or more good values. This seems to be the most problematic aspect of balancing life. It involves ranking priorities.

I have watched with interest the sacrifices that Olympic athletes make in order to compete for a gold medal. One world-class snowboarder lived in a camper on the back of his truck so he could compete. Often the sacrifice involves family. A rower who was disqualified because his boat crossed into a competitor's lane questioned whether the sacrifices he had made were really worth it. He said that he put his life on hold and missed half his daughter's life in order to compete at the Olympics. When he was disqualified, he had to grapple with the fact that he had made significant sacrifices to get to the Olympics but had not achieved his goal of a gold medal. I wonder if a medal would have made the sacrifices worth it. Certainly, the rower would have had a payoff, but at what cost?

It is important to realize that when we talk about priorities, it will usually be a painful discussion. Making something a high priority means that we will dedicate time, effort, money, and other resources to it and not to other things. Yet, this needs to be done if one is to lean into a purpose that is of value. It is a recipe for imbalance if we do not recognize that in making a fixed commitment to achieve an important goal we also need to reduce commitments in other areas.

Imbalanced Situations

Some situations naturally seem to lead to imbalance. A high-pressure job with high visibility and expectations can often create imbalance. Going back to school after being in the workforce, or parenting a young family can also produce imbalance. Imbalance is also experienced in times of loss or transition. The point is that these types of situations almost inevitably lead to imbalance. When a person is able to anticipate imbalance, they are then able to plan pro-actively to reduce or negate the impact of imbalance.

There are several things we can do to minimize imbalance. First, we should reduce commitments early rather than waiting until we are in crisis. It may feel like we are being disloyal when we drop commitments, but it is better to reduce commitments at logical end points than to leave in the middle of a term when others are depending on you. Often the hard decisions are the best decisions.

The second thing to do is negotiate how you will manage the situation with stakeholders ahead of time. If the stakeholders are your family, discuss with them the implications of the challenge facing you. Consult with others who have been through similar situations. Try to anticipate problems in advance and identify solutions that will make the challenge tolerable.

A third recommendation, if the challenging situation is going to last a significant amount of time, is to break the journey into stages and re-balance at intervals. Several of my friends have gone on to do PhDs and doctoral programs. This has had a significant impact on their families. By breaking the journey into pieces and preplanning balancing activities along the way, they have been able to manage the challenge in a more positive way.

Finally, recognize that living an imbalanced life over a long period of time can lead to an inaccurate awareness of what constitutes healthy balance. A person can get used to living an imbalanced life and this ongoing level of imbalance creates a 'new normal.' This new normal then becomes the benchmark for balance. If you are constantly living one step away from a crisis this probably applies to you. Pushing too hard for a long period of time can lead to significant consequences. That is why burnout can happen without people realizing what is happening. By constantly adjusting their new normal to a higher and higher pace, people lose an appropriate awareness of where their balance benchmark should be.

Where are you at with this balance issue? Do you feel balanced or do you need rebalance? Have you developed habits that have created a dangerous new normal?

Are you taking a balanced approach?

The question we began with helps keep us aware of our need to maintain balance in a complex world. It also helps us make balanced decisions and recognize that if we neglect key aspects of life we will likely be thrown off-balance.

One of the most significant areas we need to balance is the energy drain that comes as we live life. Hopefully this next tool will help you evaluate your situation in order to make appropriate changes.

Energy Dashboard

One of the most helpful gauges on my personal dashboard is related to energy levels. Like the speedometer, it is a point-in-time gauge. In other words, the energy dashboard reflects how I am living at a particular point in time. Energy levels change over time. By watching my energy levels, I am able to identify when I need to rebalance.

The energy dashboard has a large gauge in the middle of the work sheet. The first step is to identify your overall energy levels. Where are they right now? Are you running on fumes or do you have lots in your tank? Mark your current status on the Overall Energy Level gauge.

Next, use the other gauges to determine what areas are draining you. You will notice that these gauges differ from the Overall Energy Level gauge. They are designed to determine whether that particular life function is draining a person's energy or conversely, infusing energy back into a person's life. I have left one gauge open for you to choose an area of life that is not represented by the other gauges. If one or more of the others do not fit, simply change them to reflect your situation.

What aspects of life are causing the most drain? Obviously the areas that have the greatest drain should be assessed and steps taken to rebalance. In some cases, such as work, drain is a given and one needs to manage it well. It may not be realistic to make large changes in your workplace, but a careful review may reveal small adjustments that could make a world of difference. If every major area of your life is draining you, then you may be headed for a crisis. Take the time to re-balance as needed.

Stinson Wellness Model

ENERGY DASHBOARD

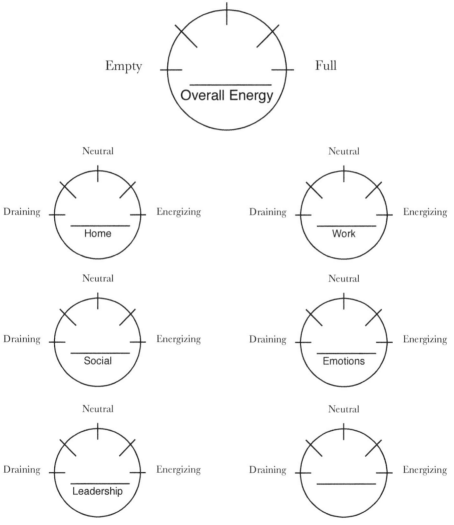

Figure 4

DISCUSSION FOUR: WORLDVIEW
What Do You Really Believe?

The Blind Men and the Elephant
John Godfrey Saxe (1816-1887)

It was six men of Indostan
To learning much inclined,
Who went to see the Elephant
(Though all of them were blind),
That each by observation
Might satisfy his mind.

The First approached the Elephant,
And happening to fall
Against his broad and sturdy side,
At once began to bawl:
"God bless me! but the Elephant
Is very like a wall!"

The Second, feeling of the tusk,
Cried, "Ho! what have we here
So very round and smooth and sharp?
To me 'tis mighty clear
This wonder of an Elephant
Is very like a spear!"

The Third approached the animal,
And happening to take
The squirming trunk within his hands,
Thus boldly up and spake:
"I see," quoth he, "the Elephant
Is very like a snake!"

The Fourth reached out his eager hand,
And felt about the knee.
"What most this wondrous beast is like
Is mighty plain," quoth he,
"Tis clear enough the Elephant
Is very like a tree!"

The Fifth, who chanced to touch the ear,
Said: "E'en the blindest man
Can tell what this resembles most;
Deny the fact who can,
This marvel of an Elephant
Is very like a fan!"

The Sixth no sooner had begun
About the beast to grope,
Then, seizing on the swinging tail
That fell within his scope,
"I see," quoth he, "the Elephant
Is very like a rope!"

And so these men of Indostan
Disputed loud and long,
Each in his own opinion
Exceeding stiff and strong,
Though each was partly in the right,
And all were in the wrong!

MORAL
So oft in theologic wars,
The disputants, I ween,
Rail on in utter ignorance
Of what each other mean,
And prate about an Elephant
Not one of them has seen! (Saxe, 1873, pp. 135-136)

Like the six blind men, each of us has a personal worldview that helps us interpret our world. Every day you and I make decisions, intentionally or automatically and without thinking, based on our personal worldview. And like the differing interpretations the blind men had of the elephant, we all see the world somewhat differently. Consequently, clarifying the characteristics of our personal worldview and recognizing the patterns of thinking that we typically use is worthwhile because with greater awareness, we gain a better understanding of how we interact with the elements of life that make up our worlds.

What do you really believe?

This discussion begins with a question, but it is different from the four pillars in that a person's worldview is the foundation the pillars stand upon. Unless the four pillars of wellness are based on a firm foundation developed by intentional thought and a clear understanding of who we are, we tend to float along with the tides and currents of culture. The task of this chapter is to help us identify what we believe so that we can build on that foundation to create greater congruence and consistency in our lives.

Alvin Toffler is credited as stating, "Every person carries in his head a mental model of the world - a subjective representation of external reality" (Sire, 2004, p. 23). He is right, we all have a picture in our mind of how the world works, what is important and how things fit together. Aerts, et al. (2007), state that "a worldview seeks to clarify the place of humanity in the world and to provide insight into the most significant relations humans have with this world, both theoretically and practically" (p. 17). As a result the concept of a worldview involves both individual perspectives as well as global considerations and are consequently difficult to articulate.

"The construction of world views is not an easy enterprise. … Instead of one view of the whole, shared by the members of a bounded collectivity, there now exist in our international world very divergent and competitive conceptions and life styles. We do not interact with one culture, but with many cultures, and even with subcultures and fragments of cultures. The individual is forced to select his or her own future life, having to choose between the enormous numbers of possibilities offered" (Aerts et al., 2007, p. 7).

At this point, we need to stop, stretch, and reflect a little. Here is a brief summary of where we have been. We have discussed two fairly straightforward questions that help us live well:

Does this take you in the direction you want to go?
Are you using a balanced approach?

These two questions prompt us to ask the next one:

What do you really believe?

All three questions are interconnected. Both purpose and balance are directed by what you believe about yourself and how you interact with the world around you. As a young university student I recognized that though I was very interested in architecture, it involved a lot of math, which I hated. I didn't think that I could succeed in architecture for that reason and consequently did not seriously consider that option. My perspective on life - my strengths and weaknesses - helped to dictate decisions related to my purpose. Discussions with my father helped me to identify that I wanted to work with people and the belief that a career working with people was a definite possibility influenced me to choose my major. These seemingly small but important thought processes have factored significantly into who I have become. They were decisions rooted in my personal worldview - my identity and understanding of my place in the world.

As a result, it is important to articulate the value and belief systems that influence how we live. We need to identify what is meaningful and what 'living well' means to us. Understanding your personal worldview helps to articulate why you have chosen your purpose(s) and why you choose to balance life the way you do.

Actions

> All the world's a stage,
> And all the men and women merely players;
> They have their exits and their entrances,
> And one man in his time plays many parts, ...
> (Shakespeare, 2008, p. 78)

Each of us lives life in front of others. We are actors in an unscripted play and we all feel that we are the stars of the show. Our understanding of each other is generally based on a self-centered perspective. Psychologists call this egocentric. In other words, the play as we experience it revolves around our experiences. If we get hurt, we feel the pain more than anyone else. If someone else gets hurt, we respond to their pain with empathy based on our past experiences. It is normal for people to interpret life based on their own personal experiences.

Our actions flow from how we understand life as interpreted through our personal worldview. This is where our inner life becomes public and impacts others in the communities in which we participate.

Actions can be observed. They are a part of a person's lifestyle. For example, you can compare how a person acts in a group with how they act one-on-one with you. You can also take note of the activities the person is involved in, such as sports teams, professional associations, or political parties. You may also observe the relationships they have with those who know them well, how they treat their family and the type of work ethic they exhibit. And if you watch carefully, you will begin to see a person's priorities in their spending habits. Lifestyle is the outer expression of the person within. Even when people try to hide who they are, we are often able to sense that they are not being genuine and become keenly aware of the inconsistencies in their lives. The same is true when others observe us.

Living consistently from the inside out is an indicator of living well. But this can be complicated. A person may live consistently from the inside out and still be misunderstood by people if those around them do not share similar values. Despite these challenges, living well is possible if a person has a well-developed personal worldview based on a strong set of values and beliefs.

A factor that adds to the complexity of a personal worldview is the fact that each of us belongs to multiple groups at a time. Each group, whether a workplace, a squash league, a church group, or a family, has its own set of values and expectations that determine how the group views the world and interprets actions. It is through these lenses that group members create meaning. The feedback we get from those around us, particularly from groups we are rooted in, encourages or discourages certain actions, depending on the collective worldview.

Consequently, our internal lives are not merely personal in nature. We live our lives in relation to others on the stage of life. There is a feedback loop from those we live with that provides commentary on how we are living.

If we observe our lifestyles and look for patterns, we can discover a lot about who we are becoming, what we believe, and the influences that affect us. The following concepts will help us understand some of the dynamics that impact our belief systems: worldview, gap, and expectations.

Worldview Origins

Worldview is a concept that Wilhelm Dilthey, a German philosopher, promoted. He identified two aspects of worldview. The first he called *Weltbild* or "world picture," which arises from one's *Lebenswelt* or "life world." This concept is similar to our current understanding of culture. For Dilthey, we are in some respects, products of our culture - how we were raised and the values within that environment. The second concept he referred to as *Weltanshauung* or "worldview" (Holmes, 1983, pp. 31-32). In contrast to the idea of "world picture," Dilthey was articulating that we each have an individual view of the world where elements may or may not match the cultural norm. The challenge is for people to find their unique identity and at the same time to recognize that where there are competing perspectives between a world picture (culture) and worldview (personal perspective) that dissonance may result.

In this discussion, world picture (Weltbild) will be referred to as a group's *collective worldview*, while worldview (Weltanshauung) will be identified as a *personal worldview*. The next sections will define the terms, identify areas where conflict may arise and help us understand how to manage the resulting dissonance.

Personal Worldview

Everyone has a personal worldview, even if they cannot articulate it. We all make decisions based on a personal framework or point of view that has a set of assumptions that may be held subconsciously. As a result, personal worldviews have many hidden aspects that need to be discovered that are intensely personal (Sire, 2004, p. 107).

Personal worldviews direct decision making and action. They reflect what a person honestly believes. Developing a personal worldview is a journey in which a person articulates what they believe and how those beliefs impact their lifestyle decisions. People who live well have taken the time to clarify their beliefs and build consistency between various aspects of life.

Phillip Johnson, a professor at Berkeley, provides the following helpful explanation related to the concept of worldview:

"… understanding how worldviews are formed, and how they guide or confine thought, is the essential step toward understanding everything else. Understanding worldview is a bit like trying to see the lens of one's own eye. We do not ordinarily see our own worldview, but we see everything else by looking through it. Put simply, our worldview is the window by which we view the world, and decide, often subconsciously, what is real and important, or unreal and unimportant. … Our worldview governs our thinking even when – or especially when – we are unaware of it" (Pearcey, 2005, p. 11).

A major process of learning to live well is to identify and articulate your personal worldview. A worldview is a system of thinking that helps to interpret events and find meaning in our lives. It may be quite disjointed and inconsistent or well articulated. Because a personal worldview encompasses how we understand all of life, some aspects of a worldview will be well developed, while others will not. The more cohesive and articulate a person's worldview, the easier it is to live intentionally and consistently.

A person may have very strong political views and organize their vote and donations around that particular point of view. Yet in other areas of life they may be far less intentional. They may not have an opinion on what sailboat is the best one to buy because they do not live on a lake and have no interest in sailing. This illustrates that there are often very natural variations in worldview development because of the variety of life experiences.

A person experiences dissonance when they say they value or believe something but their lifestyle does not reflect that value or belief. For example, a person may have very strong beliefs about fair payment for products that come from third-world countries, so they pay more for fair-trade coffee. They may, however, find it more difficult to be as consistent with large-ticket items. Ultimately, the strength of a person's value or belief is tested by whether it is reflected in their lifestyle. Do they actually make decisions based on their stated worldview? If a person is unable to act on a value or belief that is deemed to be important, they will experience dissonance.

Worldviews help us find meaning within the context of our environments, but they are seldom neatly packaged paradigms that provide all the answers we will ever need. While it is important to strive to develop an understanding of our personal worldview, we also need to recognize that we do not have to be philosophers to develop thinking patterns that allow us to live consistently in our inside and outside worlds.

What is your personal worldview? Perhaps no one has asked you this question before, so don't be too upset if you do not have a clear answer. Begin by noting things you value and watch how you make decisions. What process do you use to make key decisions? Do your values and lifestyle match? What values and beliefs actually shape your lifestyle?

Collective Worldviews

In contrast to personal worldviews that are unique to each person, collective worldviews are thought frameworks that dictate how individual groups operate. Collective worldviews are found in all kinds of groups. For example, your workplace has a collective worldview. It may be formal (written in the form of policies and procedures) or informal (certain things are frowned on or discouraged). Aspects of collective worldviews may also come to us through folklore and stories. Think of one person who should not be crossed or challenged in an organization with whom you are affiliated. How did you find out about this person? Did a colleague tell you a story about how they mistreated someone else in the past? Did you pass the information on to others?

Sports teams also have collective worldviews. They value certain ways of being. Hockey players are expected to come to the aid of and fight for their star players if the other team becomes too aggressive. Toughness is expected and rewarded. Competitive teams value wins and first place. Second place is not valued and those who come in second place are sometimes referred to as the "first looser."

John Grisham (2000), in his book entitled *A Painted House*, wrote a wonderful story about the lives of a cotton-farming family in the South. The central character is a seven-year-old boy who observes the lives of people in his community, which included seasonal laborers hired to help with the harvest. One passage in the book illustrates the difference in the collective worldviews of two churches in the small town of Black Oak:

> "The line between Baptists and Methodists was never straight and true. Their worship was slightly different, with the ritual of sprinkling little babies being their most flagrant deviation from the Scriptures, as we saw things. And they didn't meet as often, which, of course, meant that they were not as serious about their faith. Nobody met as much as us Baptists. We took great pride in constant worship. Pearl Watson, my favorite Methodist, said she'd like to be a Baptist, but that she just wasn't physically able" (p. 296).

What groups are you affiliated with? What are their values? How do the values of one organization complement or conflict with others? How do the values of these collective worldviews conflict with your personal values?

Families also have certain ways of operating. Luke, the seven year old, explained to his mother what happened in the cotton field one day:

"I think Tally and Cowboy like each other," I said, and immediately felt lighter.

"Is that so?" she said with a smile, as if I didn't know much because I was a kid. Then her smile slowly vanished as she considered this. I wondered if she, too, knew something about the secret romance.

"Yes ma'am."

"And what makes you think this?"

"I caught them in the cotton patch this mornin'."

"What were they doing?" she asked, seeming a little frightened that maybe I'd seen something I shouldn't have.

"I don't know, but they were together."

"Did you see them?"

I told her the story. ... She absorbed it and seemed genuinely astounded.

"What were they doin', Mom?"

"I don't know. You didn't see anything, did you?"

"No ma'am. Do you think they were kissin'?"

"Probably," she said quickly.

She reached for the ignition again and said, "Oh, well, I'll talk to your father about it."

We drove away in a hurry. After a moment or two I really couldn't tell if I felt any better. She told me many times that little boys shouldn't keep secrets from their mothers. But every time I confessed one, she was quick to shrug it off and tell my father what I told her" (Grisham, 2000, pp. 287-289).

The worldview in this conversation exposes that while little boys are not to keep secrets, there are plenty of secrets woven into the fabric of this family. The town, too, held many secrets that townspeople tried to uncover, often adding to the many rumors.

Your family culture and background may be very different from this illustration, but you have a family background with its own unique patterns. If you can identify the patterns of your family worldview, it will shed light on the origins of your personal worldview. It is common for us to act in certain ways without understanding how we came to have this behavior embedded in our personalities, so take time to reflect on your family heritage.

It is especially important to be aware of your family history – not to point fingers at anyone, but simply to understand where you have come from. There is often a temptation to blame parents or siblings for issues from the past. These certainly need to be dealt with, but I encourage you to shift your focus and look to the future. Don't let the past dictate who you will become. Dream. Live with intentionality and become the person you hope to be. Make good decisions and align your life based on what you believe.

The point of this discussion is that we live concurrently in multiple environments with differing collective worldviews that may or may not synchronize with each other or with our personal values and beliefs. Sorting through these patterns and recognizing where there is conflict is a valuable exercise that helps to inform our thought patterns.

Living well, then, includes a complex challenge to synthesize one's personal worldview (as complete or incomplete as it is) with the various collective worldviews represented in a person's life. To find peace and tranquility in a complex culture takes a lot of work. Even though we might strive to have a very clear and concise worldview, personal worldviews are usually messy and inconsistent. Acknowledge the mess, but don't get discouraged. If you keep working to clarify your personal worldview, it will happen over time.

Gaps between Expectations and Reality

Gaps are created when parts of our worlds do not synchronize very well. We all have gaps and inconsistencies in our lives. Some gaps are internal, while others are external. Gaps are created when expectations and reality do not match.

An internal gap is created when a person does not consistently live out their values and beliefs. The result is dissonance. If the dissonance is relatively minor, a person can live with it for a long period of time. But if the gap is related to a significant aspect of a person's life, they will employ various techniques to alleviate the effect of the gap. Over time, if the gap is not addressed adequately, the dissonance can become so intense that a person may make a major change in their belief system or lifestyle in order to reduce the gap.

Gaps can also be external. An external gap is created when a person does not meet the expectations of another person or group of people. External gaps are often found in the family and work life. Gaps caused by differing expectations are common to all parts of life. By tracking expectations, a person is better able to identify gaps that emerge and understand the resulting behavior of themselves and others.

We need to acknowledge the gaps in our lives. They are normal. By working to minimize gaps where we have strong convictions or well-articulated perspectives, we are able to move toward greater internal consistency.

Expectations

We all have expectations of others and ourselves. Typically expectations are set high and often go unmet. Being realistic about expectations helps us close some of our gaps.

It is important that we carefully explore where expectations come from and whether we want to continue to hold on to them or not. There is some merit to Homer Simpson's philosophy of lowering expectations to the point that you are never disappointed, but it is probably not the best approach to life. One of my bosses pointed out one day that some things are not worth doing well. I considered him to be a very competent and thorough person, so I knew he had put some thought behind this statement. His comment illuminates the idea that we need to use priorities to direct our lives. Things that have a lower priority may warrant less time and energy. We need to put the most time and effort into the things that are most important.

Expectations and the roles they play differ from culture to culture. It is worth noting that the collective worldviews of two different cultures may dictate different actions in similar situations. What is expected in one culture may be frowned on in another. Cultural expectations differ widely, and the script that supports the logic of the cultural pattern also differs between cultures. It is important to recognize that the values and patterns of each culture have strengths and weaknesses. Since we tend to judge others from the perspective of our home culture, let's be open to the idea that other cultures may inform us in ways our culture does not. We also need to be aware of any inconsistencies outsiders may see in our culture.

Choice

A central assumption related to living well is that we have the opportunity to make choices about many things. It is true that some people have greater opportunity to make certain decisions than others, but most of us do not realize how much choice we really have.

In his book entitled *Man's Search for Meaning*, Viktor Frankl (1959) wrote about his experience as a prisoner in a concentration camp during World War II.

> "We who lived in concentration camps can remember the men who walked through the huts comforting others, giving away their last piece of bread. They may have been few in number, but they offer sufficient proof that everything can be taken from a man but one thing: the last of the human freedoms—to choose one's attitude in any given set of circumstances, to choose one's own way. And there were always choices to make. Every day, every hour, offered the opportunity to make a decision, a decision which determined whether you would or would not submit to those powers which threatened to rob you of your very self, your inner freedom; which determined whether or not you would become the plaything of circumstance, renouncing freedom and dignity to become molded into the form of the typical inmate. ... Even though conditions such as lack of sleep, insufficient food and various mental stresses may suggest that the inmates were bound to react in certain ways, in the final analysis it becomes clear that the sort of person the prisoner became was the result of an inner decision, and not the result of camp influences alone" (pp. 86-87).

Even in dire situations, people have the opportunity to choose their attitude and how they interpret events. The ability to choose is an important aspect of internal motivation. How many of your decisions are motivated from within? How many have been dictated externally, by the environment and people around you?

What do I really believe?

The primary premise of this book is that we need to make wise decisions that align with who we are. We began this discussion by asking: What do you really believe? As we find answers, we begin to identify who we are and then can align our beliefs and lifestyle to live authentically.

DISCUSSION FIVE: CONGRUENCE
Do your actions reflect your values and beliefs?

The term congruent is defined as being "in agreement or harmony" or "identical in form; coinciding exactly when superimposed" (Woolf, 1980, p. 236). With regard to our lives, congruence is evidenced when our actions match our values and beliefs.

Congruence is related to a maturing identity that is based on a cohesive personal worldview. As a person builds their identity around the core of who they are, they become stronger and more centered. Whereas purpose is about direction and movement, congruence is about meaning and fulfillment. We can be very active and successful (purpose and direction) and yet not find meaning in life. Because congruence is based on each person's personal value and belief system, congruence will look somewhat different for everyone.

Defining your identity

As was noted in the wellbeing literature, living well is connected to identifying our true self (our daimon). When I was in university I thought I knew myself reasonably well. I didn't know that there was a true self to discover. In retrospect, I had a lot to learn. Looking back I can now begin to see some of the significant threads that are woven into my psyche that I was somewhat unaware of when I was younger. As a young man, I often developed my identity instinctively and could not explain how or what was driving me. I tended to know how I felt about things, but not why I felt that way. Over the years, by observing my tendencies and analyzing my history I have become much more aware of who I am and I can articulate it far more succinctly—I have uncovered my true self and have developed my own voice.

I'm not sure that there is a specific process for discovering your true self other than deep reflection and observation. But I have come to believe that we need to discover who we really are down deep, and this involves work and time. It is challenging to discover one's true self and then to develop congruence based on that understanding.

Our identities shift somewhat as we go through life. Yes, to an extent a person's personality remains the same, but as circumstances change, we redefine ourselves. Marriage redefined who I was. Likewise, having kids changed how I viewed myself, shifting my identity yet again. Changes in health, at work, in family life, or in any other major area can cause us to redefine our identity. As a result, identities tend to shift over the course of a lifetime. Living congruently reflects this journey.

Congruence also has to do with aligning multiple areas of life. We need to align our belief systems with other aspects of life, such as our natural abilities and talents. This causes us to look inward to discover the deepest expression of who we are as unique human beings.

I recall making the decision *not* to become a doctor because I did not like blood and guts. I grew up in Africa and had the opportunity, as did many of my peers, to watch surgical procedures. I never took that opportunity; I was not interested. But something deep inside me motivates me to create. I love new ideas, putting ideas into new forms, designing things, and creating art. And I can track this interest from a very young age. As a child I loved to draw. At about the age of eight I remember trying to design something I had never seen before, but what to day is known as a motor home. I dreamed of parking it in a field close to our home in Africa and watching wild animals at night. In university, I was driven to write something new or find different angles when writing papers, and I intentionally tried to think differently. The urge to create emanates from deep within my soul. When I recognized this and applied it to my career path, I began to look for opportunities that allow me to express creativity in my work. This perspective replaced an earlier goal of climbing the corporate ladder. And it has led to greater meaning and higher satisfaction levels at work.

Stinson Wellness Model
FINDING YOUR SWEET SPOT
(LUCADO 2005, P. 147-178)

Things that I have enjoyed doing:	Age when this occurred:

Figure 5

Take time to fill this out several times. Think back to when you were a child, when you were a teenager and then as an adult. What activities have you found most fulfilling? Look for patterns that might lead you to identify your sweet spot.

How sucessful was I? (1low, 10 high)	What made me successful?

Figure 5

An author, Max Lucado, uses a set of exercises designed to help readers identify themes that run throughout their lives, from childhood to adulthood. The exercise helps identify passions and giftedness. He recommends that we watch for times in the past when we have been successful and enjoyed what we were doing. I suggest that you do this too. (Figure 4) Once you have identified some of these times, ask what made you successful and why it felt so satisfying. By looking for patterns that began early in life, we can get a sense of what our "sweet spot" might be. Knowing our sweet spot allows us to look for future opportunities where our strengths and passions can be harnessed. Look deeply at who you are. Begin to align your lifestyle with who you are on the inside.

Meaning and resilience

Living from the inside out enhances our ability to live passionately and authentically. Meaning flows from within. We find meaning when we are able to use our talents and passions to benefit others and by being true to one's self as we live congruently based a cohesive personal worldview.

When a person lives an aligned life, they are able to be far more resilient and less concerned about what others think. Resilience allows people to make mistakes and still have high self-esteem. Resilient people are able to admit their weaknesses and own their struggles. At the same time, they understand their strengths and seek to use them for the benefit of others. This sense of identity and comfort in our own skins allows for the learning mindset that Carol Dweck believes develops success. She states: "The passion for stretching yourself and sticking to it, even (or especially) when it's not going well, is the hallmark of the growth mindset. This is the mindset that allows people to thrive during some of the most challenging times of their lives" (2007, p. 7). Having a growth mindset, combined with a strong sense of congruence, allows for great learning and authenticity as people progress through life.

Discovery

I recently went through some goal-planning sheets I made in my thirties. Some goals I can check off because I have fulfilled them, but many of the goals I have not yet achieved are still the same. What I have realized is that these goals and dreams are connected to the core of who I am. One dream was to build a house that reflects my identity and creativity. In the process of renovating our home a few years ago, we were able to really make it 'ours.' My wife and I both feel as though it reflects our personalities. The desire to build a home that is unique and personal is really reflective of my value for creativity. My dreams reflect my values. My journey of wellness has led me to discover the core of who I am. As I continue to discover more about myself, I am better able to live congruently.

Peace

Whereas the world around us creates all kinds of divergent pressures and 'noise,' living from the inside fosters peace. That is not to say we will not encounter struggles, but rather, when we do we will have something much more solid to base our lives on. I encourage you to understand the core of who you are and base your decisions on that understanding. As you do you will find greater inner peace.

This book has intentionally steered away from religion and has focused on helping people to develop their own personal value and belief systems. It should be noted, however, that philosophy and religion both attempt to answer the deep questions of life. Even though we don't think that deeply on a day-to-day basis, many of the assumptions that guide our thinking originate in those two fields.

There is a sense in which delving deeply into major questions of life can become so abstract that it can become confusing. Having said that, I think we all should carefully evaluate what we believe to ensure that we have actually chosen those beliefs. In addition, I do not think that just because a person can argue their position well because they have a cohesive worldview, means that they will find greater inner peace. Nor does inner peace rest with those who seem to have everything in life. There is a quality to inner peace that seems to go far beyond cognitive process, wealth or power. My encouragement is to search for what provides you with inner peace and contentment.

Do your actions reflect your values and beliefs?

Congruence is built on a person's developing worldview. We can work on congruence as we continue to articulate our worldview. Do you feel free enough to allow your inner self to rise to the surface? What changes might you consider to bring greater alignment between your inner desires and the outward expression of them in your lifestyle? Have you dedicated time, effort, and money to your passions? By regularly reflecting on questions like these, we are challenged to live from the inside out.

DISCUSSION SIX: SUSTAINABILITY
Can you do this long term?

The concept of sustainability is often understood in relation to the environment. We use less paper in packaging so that we do not throw away as much garbage. By using energy-saving light bulbs, we do not waste power. Pollution in the air, water, and environment is reduced so that the earth is not damaged. These are just a few examples of environmental issues that the term sustainability references.

The same concept can be applied to our personal lives. What behaviors might we limit so that we do not damage good habits that assist us to live well? What life adjustments will help us to live longer? What emotional stressors do we need to manage well in order to enjoy long term mental health? Are we pacing ourselves physically to go the distance?

Balance and sustainability are linked. Living a balanced life focuses on balancing the various elements in life so that we are not neglecting anything important. When we live balanced lives we are much more likely to be able to live sustainable lives. Sustainability is found when we are able to live well for long periods of time without compromising health and vitality.

To live well, we need to address the concept of sustainability on various levels, but in order to simplify this discussion I will identify and discuss a few aspects of sustainability that are of primary importance.

Energy – Two Sides of One Coin

Side One

One side of personal sustainability has to do with managing energy drain. Experiencing sustainability is about living within our means – emotionally, physically, socially, spiritually, and financially.

We understand that living within our financial means requires that we limit spending according to our income. In the same way, we need to balance cost (drain) with income (revitalizing activities and people). The dashboard exercise in the balance chapter was a snapshot of your energy levels at a point in time. Sustainability looks at energy expense over a long period of time. If people expend more energy than they take in, they begin drawing on their reserves. If this trend continues, they will find themselves in a deficit position and have to take out a loan; they will take time, energy and resources from other areas of life to manage the deficit. These short term loans may solve the problem initially, but over time they can have a significant negative impact on an individual's well being. So one side of the coin has to do with identifying the energy cost over time.

Side Two

The other side of the coin is related to replenishing the energy we spend. Energy and renewal are created when we do enjoyable things that we are passionate about. In addition, energy is increased when we are with people we enjoy and with whom we share similar values and activities. These are people we can trust to support and understand us when needed. They accept and love us as we are. Because of this, we can laugh and cry together; we can play games and work together.

It is important to realize that what recharges one person may be quite different from what recharges another. One person might want to recharge by going to a party, while another might want to go for a long walk in the woods. Since recharging is personal in nature, take the time to figure out what you find rejuvenating. By intentionally building these things into your schedule, you will be able to live a more sustainable lifestyle.

Rest is a common way to recharge. What does this look like? It could mean that you schedule a golf game with people you like once a month. Or it could be as simple as blocking off time for a nap or eight hours of sleep each night. In many religions, the idea of setting time apart for rest and meditation is recommended. Sabbath, as it is referred to in the Bible, is the practice of reserving one day of the week for rest. Regardless of your belief system, regular rest is a good habit to cultivate. Build rest into your schedule.

Sometimes I feel guilty and selfish for scheduling renewing events into my calendar, but more and more I am convinced that I need to be very strategic in protecting this side of the coin. I have seen too many people burn out and get themselves into difficult situations because they neglected sustainability. The consequences, at times, have been tragic.

Sustainability, then, is not about getting rid of challenges in life. Rather, it is about finding a way to manage challenges well so that we do not suffer long term negative effects. Sustainable living is based on a realistic, long term approach to life that is grounded in our identity and belief system.

Personal Sustainability

Sustainability questions must be answered individually. We all have different thresholds and tolerances. Just because another person seems to get by on six hours of sleep a night does not mean you can too. Some people have lots of energy, while others do not. One person may love studying, while another may need to be outside and moving. The point is that we are all different, so we must base sustainability on who we are as individuals.

In this regard, sustainability is also based on a person's passions and strengths. A person expends less energy when they work from an area of strength, compared with when they work from an area of weakness. When much of a person's work time is spent in areas of weakness, they are more likely to encounter burnout and other stress related illnesses.

I have never been very good at math. When I grab a calculator to try and solve a math problem, others have already solved it in their heads. Things that require math cause me stress. What is complex for me is simple for others. As a result, I expend a great deal of energy trying to complete math projects properly. Much to my amazement, there are people who enjoy work that involves math - and they are far better at it than me. I have learned that to manage my life well I need to find ways to be involved in areas where I have strengths to offer. This has helped me to be more successful and has allowed me to give more in my workplace.

By identifying our strengths and weaknesses we are able to determine how to maximize the energy we expend. Take a look at your life. What drains you? What aspects of life come naturally? Are you working from areas of strength or areas of weakness? If you can, write down your strengths and ask yourself what you might change to use them more effectively.

Clarifying priorities and beliefs also develops sustainability. As we noted in the worldview chapter, we often live with tensions and gaps. When we minimize gaps and develop greater congruence between our internal and external lives, we reduce energy expense. The process of aligning one's life produces greater sustainability. Consequently, worldview and congruence provide an important context for making sustainable decisions.

Vitality

Vitality is an outcome of living well. People often picture wellness as tanned twenty-year-old athletes playing volleyball on the beach (with a cooler of beer on ice to quench their thirsts after the game). But living well is not just about youth and health. A helpful way to think about wellness is to define wellness as *living with vitality within the context of one's personal limitations*. People who live well do not allow their limitations to dictate what they can and cannot do. Nor do they follow a formula or imitate others. Instead, they adapt to changes by seeing modifiers instead of limiters; they maximize their strengths and abilities; and look to values and beliefs they have chosen for guidance.

My father-in-law, who lived into his mid-eighties, is a good example of a person who lived with vitality right to the end of his life. Despite health setbacks that limited his physical activity, he continued to volunteer at his church and various other places. He also stayed connected with friends, family, and even the nurses in the hospital. He always had a smile on his face, a twinkle in his eye and a story to tell. On his deathbed, he was still in contact with friends in India where he spent much of his adult life. Dad lived well despite the limitations at the end of his life.

Do you allow yourself to be defined by your limitations? Many of us do not live well because we allow a limitation, big or small, to keep us from living meaningful lives. We see brick walls rather than doors. At times, we define wellbeing in terms of what we do not have in comparison with others. Do not compare yourself with others. There will always be people who have things you want. Note, too, that there will be people who look at you and wish they had what you have. Choose to have a positive attitude and focus on things you are passionate about and you will live with vitality.

Draining People

Depending on your personality, you will find certain people more draining than others. Acknowledge this and identify that those people take a lot out of you. Keep in mind, however, that we are on this earth to contribute to others, which is draining. The goal is not to eliminate energy drain, but to manage it.

The first step in managing draining people is to become aware of who they are and what causes the drain. Put some thought into structures that you might put in place to limit the amount of drain they can place on you. I have people in my life that I will not meet with unless they book an appointment in advance. I also set a limit on the length of time scheduled for each visit. This helps me to manage the drain.

Identifying people who recharge you is as important as understanding what drains you. Intentionally schedule these people into your life on a regular basis. We should aim to balance the amount of drain with the people and activities needed to recharge us.

Assignment

When we discussed balance, you took the time to fill out the Energy Dashboard. That was a way to identify your energy levels at that point in time. If you were to use the same exercise every month, you could plot your energy levels over a year. (You may want to do that if the following discussion and exercise are difficult to grasp.) Since sustainability is about healthy living over a long period of time, it is important to track energy levels over time, paying specific attention to seasonal and cyclical aspects of your lifestyle.

Stinson Wellness Model
SPEED AND ENERGY OVER TIME

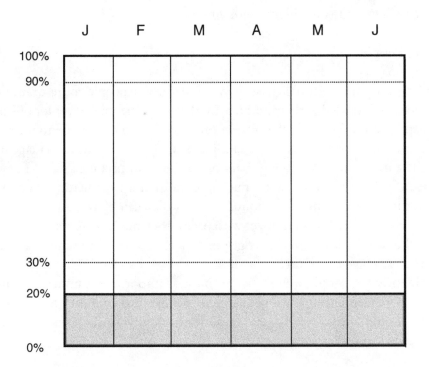

Health Zone:

Inversion Zone:

3:1 Ratio:

Recharging Ides:

Figure 6

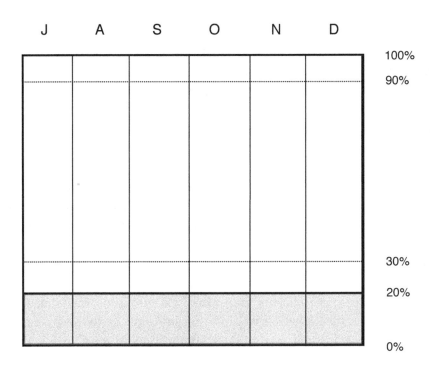

Figure 6

I have designed a worksheet that will help you track your energy levels over the course of a year and have included an explanation of how to use the form. This form has been one of the most helpful tools that I have used to help me understand my personal wellness. Please take the time to read the instructions because they include a number of new concepts that I have developed along the way.

Energy Over Time Worksheet

This worksheet represents the idea that we will gradually run out of energy if we expend more energy than we generate. The amount of drain on a battery is related to the level of use. Similarly, if you are using a lot of energy at work, you may feel significant drain over time, and it may take more time than you think is needed to recharge. Tracking energy drain over time and being proactive about recharging are critical aspects of living well.

Now take the time to graph your energy level over the last year. The vertical lines on the graph create twelve sections, which represent the twelve months of the year. The easiest way to do this is to jot down times when you felt drained (the lows). Think about what caused the drain. Think, too, about times you felt rejuvenated (the highs). Vacations often contribute to renewal. As you identify these ups and downs, note them on the worksheet in the appropriate month. When you are done, connect the dots to create a graph.

If I were to fill out the graph for July through December, the first semester of the academic year, I would begin in August with lots of energy because I would have just returned to work after a good vacation in July. But very quickly, the drain intensifies as we train student leaders and new students arrive for Orientation Week. We work long days, interact with many people, and are very focused on ensuring the functions that we are responsible for are running well. It is a high-drain season of the year. As the semester progresses, I find my energy levels continue to drop to the point that I get very tired toward the end of the semester. By charting my energy levels for several years, I realized that every year had a similar pattern and I could be more proactive in managing the drain. I now take care to place renewing activities into my schedule during and after the busy times so that I can live in a more sustainable manner.

There is a relationship between energy levels and workload. Obviously, when the workload is very high, a person's energy level drops quickly. You should already have a line on your worksheet that represents your energy level. Now go back and using different color pen, track the intensity of your workload. If your primary drain is coming from work you will find that the two lines have similar highs and lows, but that the energy level line will lag behind the workload line. This is because the work drains our energy reserves. At the beginning of the year, I can sustain a heavy workload for a limited amount of time until my energy levels begin to drop. Then I get tired and need to address the drain.

Notice that the lag also applies to rejuvenating times like vacation. It takes a certain amount of time once on vacation before the energy levels begin to pick up again. If you have experienced a heavy drain for a significant period of time, it will take a good chunk of rest before you get your energy back. This is why we need to be strategic about how we spend vacation time. Chunks of time away may produce greater energy regeneration than a day away here and there. I have noticed that it usually takes me a week of rest before my energy begins to return.

Once you have graphed your energy levels and workload, go back and try to identify what caused them to fluctuate. You might want to take another color and chart the drain from family involvement at different parts of the year. Maybe you are volunteering with an organization and there are busy times that affect your energy levels. Try to figure out what the main drivers are of the changes to your energy levels.

Let me also explain the numbers on the graph. The numbers represent critical points to watch, but are based on relationships rather than specific data. For example, I have set the healthy band at between 30% and 90%. The numbers are reference points that designate transitions that people need to keep in mind.

90%-100%

The top band is characterized by sprinting at top speed. Sprinting can only be done for short distances, takes a lot of energy and requires frequent rests. The top band is not a healthy place to live long term, but it is a place we all encounter at various points in life. The thing to remember when working at this level is that it can only be sustained for short periods of time and because it takes a great deal of energy, a person should plan to recharge after the sprint to offset the energy drain.

To offset the drain of the start of school, I now try to keep the two weekends in the middle of September free so that I can recharge. This allows me to spend time with my wife and go kayaking or camping. I encourage you to identify the times when you have to sprint. For accountants, it may be tax season. For pastors, it may be Sundays. And for farmers, it may be harvest time. Watch for your busy times and plan recovery times after each sprint.

30%-90%

The health zone is a wide band. Remember that this healthy zone is personal in nature. What might be healthy for one person may not be for another. Where people encounter physical, emotional, or mental health issues, the band will tend to be smaller. Increased health and wellbeing widens this band.

20%-30%

This is the warning zone. In my opinion, it is the most critical zone on the chart. I have noticed a lot of people are unaware of their warning signs and consequently go from health to sickness without really knowing what happened. If we become aware of our personal warning signs, we can make changes before it is too late.

Invisible Lines

Before we talk more about warning signs, I want to explain a concept I call invisible lines. One day I got a telephone call informing me that my friend's wife had left him and the children. Many of our friends jumped into action to try and avert the crisis. In the end, nothing could change her mind. Her decision was made. Upon reflection, I realized that she had made her decision to leave long before she acted on it. Some time earlier, she reached a breaking point that caused her to decide to leave. She crossed a line and none of her friends had any idea that it had happened. This incident got me thinking about hidden decision points that I call invisible lines. The problem is that we often cross lines in our personal lives that we do not see coming. At times, crossing these lines comes with significant consequences. If we were able to see the line, we would stop before crossing it. But because it is invisible, we are unaware of the significance of the decision.

I recall a time when a fellow employee confided that he would not work with one of our colleagues anymore. My friend explained that he had tried to work with this other employee and time after time found himself frustrated with the outcome. One day he had had enough. That was it. A line had been crossed and he lost respect for this colleague. The outcome was that cooperation between the two departments, represented by these two people, was virtually eliminated.

As I have become aware of this concept, I have seen many examples of invisible lines. One friend found himself on stress leave because of the great amount of stress he encountered in his workplace. His comment was, "I didn't see it coming. I thought I was doing fine."

The point of this discussion is that while these lines may be invisible the warning signs are not. If we can become aware of signs that signal we are in danger, then we have the opportunity to make changes before we cross an invisible line. The dark line at 20% on the chart represents an invisible line.

Warning Signs

A friend is married to a pilot. She thinks of warning signs using an aircraft metaphor. If an aircraft is too low, an alarm will sound to tell the pilot he needs to pull up and gain more altitude. If he does not, he may crash. In the same way, we have warning signs that alert us to a pending crash. They tell us to 'pull up' and make a significant course adjustment. By being aware of our warning signs, we can avoid a personal catastrophe.

What are warning signs? How can I recognize them? Let me give you some examples. Warning signs range from common experiences to more severe symptoms. For example, when we begin to get tired we become irritable, maybe short tempered or emotional. When we encounter stress, our stomachs knot up or we may feel heaviness in the chest. These are normally gentle reminders from our body that we need to take better care of ourselves.

105

If we ignore common warning signs we will encounter more severe symptoms. When we wake up tired even after a good eight-hour sleep, we should interpret this as a possible warning sign. Another warning sign may be when we are too tired to exercise or keep up regular routines that we normally enjoy. Over time, if we find ourselves constantly battling sickness, we should make a correction before we encounter a major or long term illness.

A colleague explained that she loves being outside walking her dogs in the beautiful natural environment surrounding her home, but sometimes when she is exhausted she does not even want to walk her dogs or be near another living being. When we begin to isolate ourselves from even our closest friends or spouses/partners we should recognize that we are experiencing a major warning sign.

My wife, Becky, has noticed that one of her warning signs is no longer enjoying things that normally replenish her. The things she usually loves to do are no longer attractive. What people or activities replenish you? When you no longer find them enjoyable, you need to take caution. Restlessness often accompanies this warning sign. You want something, but do not know exactly what that is. When I feel this way, I want to escape. I want to go somewhere to get away from problems, a place where I can focus on myself and enjoy life for a while.

Finally, a very significant warning sign is when characteristics that normally describe you are no longer evident in your life. You begin to lose the qualities that define you. By nature, I enjoy people and want to help them. I normally feel recharged when I am with people, so I know I am in the warning zone when I find myself avoiding people or hoping I do not see another person for the rest of the day. When I begin to dream about a deserted island, I know I need to recharge because I normally hate being alone. What are your warning signs? Make a list of them so that you remember to watch for them.

1%–20%

The inversion zone is the lowest level. If you drop below your healthy level and do nothing to change your energy levels, you will cross an invisible line and find yourself in significant trouble. This is when people go on stress leave or have a mental or an emotional breakdown. It is a place we do not want to end up because it usually takes a long time to recover.

The reason I call it the inversion zone is because by this point people are sick and are no longer able to be their normal selves. They move into a protective shell to promote recovery.

To illustrate this, think about when you get sick. Your body essentially says, "I have had enough and you are going to crawl into bed and sleep for a day or two." After we take care of our bodies, we begin to recover – slowly.

Similar things happen when we reach a mental or an emotional crisis. Our bodies tell us we are not living well and that we need to become very self-centered for a while in order to recharge our batteries. We are in self-protection mode until we begin to recover.

In the inversion zone we become like turtles, we pull our head and legs into the safety of the shell. When we begin to feel better and it is safe to go out again, we then stick out our necks, look around and begin moving.

In the inversion zone we are not the same people we are when we are healthy. We are self-centered because we are sick. It is our bodies' way of helping us recover. My observation is that when something breaks badly, the road to recovery is long. The better option is always to address things earlier, rather than later.

Can you do this long term?

What do you need to change to live in the healthy band? Does your alignment reflect your priorities? Have you scheduled recovery time after periods of great drain or intensity? Is part of your recovery related to spirituality? Does your soul need to heal? What do you need to do to align your life from the inside out? These questions should put you on the right track to live well, long term.

DISCUSSION SEVEN: WISE DECISION MAKING
How can I apply this to real life?

The goal of this book is to help people live with purpose, balance, congruence, and sustainability. Since each of the wellness pillars are applied personally to decisions, the wellness model allows for individualized decision making. As Waterman et al have noted, better choices are ones that align with one's true self or *daimon* (Waterman et al, 2008). Applying these four principles to decision making helps create greater intrinsic motivation.

Not too long ago, I considered a work opportunity in my field. As I contemplated whether I would apply for the job, it occurred to me to use the pillars as a template for analyzing the decision.

First, I looked at purpose. Would applying for this job take me in the direction I wanted to go? I had to look carefully at my talents and passions. I am a reasonably good administrator, but it is not my passion. The job looked as if it would include more administration. Second, the job would have provided a better opportunity for moving up the administrative ladder, which might have been nice, but my impression was it would reduce the ability to work creatively. In the end, my analysis related to purpose was that the position would not move me in the direction I wanted to go.

When I looked at balance, I recognized it would mean a move to another community. It would create imbalance for my family at a particularly strategic time in their lives. It would have also meant that Becky would have to quit working at a school she loves and find a new job in a different community. In my current role, I have a large network of valued friends and colleagues. The new job would require a lot of hard work developing friends in a new community and relationships in a new organization. Changing jobs would create significant imbalance.

As I evaluated congruence, I noted my current job offers a lot of congruence. I have been at my university for over 25 years and know how things work. For the most part, I really enjoy what I do. I recognized that a new job would mean starting all over and the work environment would likely be much less congruent than the one I currently enjoy.

Sustainability could have been better at this new job with a higher rate of pay, but it would also put me at the bottom of the seniority scale. A downturn in the economy could mean I would be one of the first people laid off. In the end, I decided not to apply for the job.

I have used this grid regularly since then to analyze key decisions as diverse as buying a car to setting goals for my department. I encourage you to try it and see if it helps you make better decisions. The following chart will walk you through the process.

Note that the goal is to live from the inside out. At the bottom of the chart is the term worldview, which includes your thinking patterns, values and beliefs. As you think through the pillars, recognize that they unify the different layers of life. Wise decision making requires a careful evaluation of what you value and how those values get expressed in your lifestyle. I hope you find it helpful.

Stinson Wellness Model

WISE DECISION MAKING

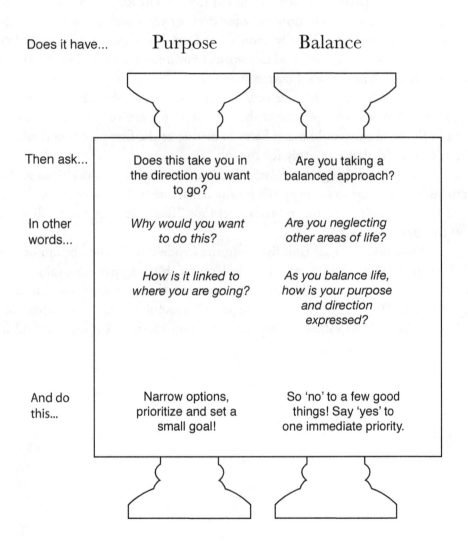

	Purpose	Balance
Does it have...		
Then ask...	Does this take you in the direction you want to go?	Are you taking a balanced approach?
In other words...	*Why would you want to do this?*	*Are you neglecting other areas of life?*
	How is it linked to where you are going?	*As you balance life, how is your purpose and direction expressed?*
And do this...	Narrow options, prioritize and set a small goal!	So 'no' to a few good things! Say 'yes' to one immediate priority.

Worldview: Values and Beliefs

Figure 7

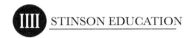 STINSON EDUCATION

Congruence   Sustainability

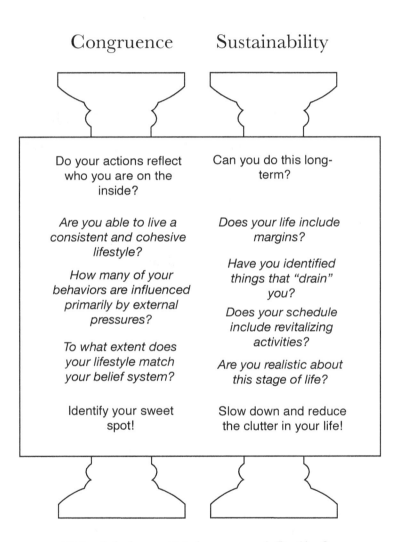

Do your actions reflect who you are on the inside?

Can you do this long-term?

Are you able to live a consistent and cohesive lifestyle?

Does your life include margins?

How many of your behaviors are influenced primarily by external pressures?

Have you identified things that "drain" you?

Does your schedule include revitalizing activities?

To what extent does your lifestyle match your belief system?

Are you realistic about this stage of life?

Identify your sweet spot!

Slow down and reduce the clutter in your life!

Worldview: Values and Beliefs

Figure 7

DISCUSSION EIGHT: WELLNESS IN SOCIETY
What can I contribute to those around me?

The discussion in this book has focused primarily on our personal lives. It is important that we take time to reflect on these things, but it is also crucial that we balance personal wellness with the obligation to contribute to society.

Early universities functioned with the understanding that one of the outcomes of a good education was that graduates would be able to contribute to society, to be good citizens. The Western world, however, has become increasingly self-centered. When it comes to wellness, it is not uncommon for people to focus primarily on themselves and their needs without much thought for others. To live well includes both managing our personal lives well and actively participating in the communities that surround us. So it is important we take time to think about our footprints in society.

Good citizens give more than they take because they understand they are a functioning part of society. For society to be better, we all must play a part. What kind of a citizen are you? How much do you take and what do you give back? Imagine if everyone gave a little more than they took. What would society look like?

Living well is very personal, but as each individual lives well and compassionately engages with society, wellness becomes the foundation for building healthy communities. Healthy people create healthy communities and healthy communities create strong societies.

I know, as I am writing, I am likely speaking to people who do give back to their communities. There is a danger of giving too much and in the process, not caring for yourself. Healthy individuals give to others, but are also able to receive from them as well. So if you are a giver, you may need to work on receiving. A part of healthy living is allowing others to give to you as they see fit. This is a challenge for me. I often turn down offers of help partly because I do not think people really want to help. It is also because I like things done a certain way. But I have come to realize that allowing someone to help me is a healthy part of living in community. It establishes a web of community, in the sense that all members of a group give and receive at certain times. My point is that if we are only giving or only taking we are not living well. It is this idea of reciprocal caring that strengthens a society.

Be a positive resource in your community. Contribute your talents and passions to others and be willing to receive from others who are also using their talents and passions to better society. As we all do our part, I believe we will be able to make a significant and positive difference in our communities.

CONCLUSION

We have discussed the pillars of wellness and how they link to the core of who we are. We have also recognized that our lifestyles reflect our inner lives. I have provided some tools to help you to assess where you have been and where you might want to go. In addition, I have encouraged you to begin to articulate your personal worldview and recognize that synchronizing it with other world-views might be a real challenge. We have talked about a lot of life.

The challenge now is to begin the journey. Where does your journey need to begin? Are you in crisis mode and need to deal with your immediate circumstances? Maybe you need to reformulate your goals? Possibly you have to say 'no' to some good things in order to rebalance and set a new direction. You may be in an incongruent situation and need to identify a way to find greater congruence. Or possibly you need to get to a more sustainable place so that you have the needed resources to engage in the journey. I encourage you to begin by taking small steps forward.

If you are not in crisis mode, you may need to revisit purpose. Take time to dream. Look deeply within. What is your heart saying to you? Listen a little. Find your soul. I like what Palmer (2000) has to say about this:

"The soul is like a wild animal – tough, resilient, savvy, self-sufficient, and yet exceedingly shy. If we want to see a wild animal, the last thing we should do is to go crashing through the woods, shouting for the creature to come out. But if we are willing to walk quietly into the woods and sit silently for an hour or two at the base of a tree, the creature we are waiting for may well emerge ..." (pp. 7-8).

I do not like silence or isolation. But being quiet and centered can happen even amidst the busyness of life if a person is intentional. It does not happen on its own, however, and it does not seem to be a natural process. That is why we often get ourselves into such a mess. Begin by finding room to quietly wait and listen.

I want to leave you with a picture of your soul – from God's perspective. Forgive me because this reflects my belief system, but I think it speaks to the nature of the soul. In *The Shack*, William P. Young (2007) uses the analogy of a shack to explain how his life was dreary and unfulfilling until he had a significant encounter with God. After looking at his life and realizing all his striving to become successful had resulted in becoming a shack that needed a complete renovation rather than a mansion everyone wanted, Young wrote the following analogy. Mack, the main character, encounters God, who looks at the yard around the shack and says:

> "… this garden is your soul. This mess is you! Together you and I, we have been working with a purpose in your heart. And it is wild and beautiful and perfectly in process. To you it seems like a mess, but to me, I see a perfect pattern emerging and growing and alive …" (p. 138).

I know I often see a mess when I look at my inner life. But the beauty in this for me is that I represent a wild, lovely mess that is growing and alive. My soul is living and, even though it is messy, it has a wild beauty embedded there. As I listen to my heart and begin to see the pattern of my soul, I can fully grow into who I am meant to be.

I do not know what your beliefs are, but I hope they provide you with the peace and joy my own give me. I hope you have the freedom to embrace the beauty and wildness of your soul.

THANKS!

Thanks for reading to the end. I trust something you have encountered will be useful. I encourage you to continue your journey to live well – whatever that looks like for you. I hope, too, that by attempting to live well, our positive influences will counteract some of the negative aspects in our societies.

YOU MAY BE INTERESTED TO KNOW

The Stinson Wellness Model is being adapted for use in business. Dr. Mark Lee, a professor of Business at Trinity Western University, and I have coauthored two articles to date.

In 2013, our journal article published in the International Journal of Strategic Management, entitled Sustaining Corporate Performance through Employee Wellbeing: Applying the Stinson Wellness Model in a Business Environment, won the Outstanding Research Paper Award from the International Academy of Business and Economics (Volume 13, Number 3, 2013).

Our 2014 journal article, published in the European Journal of Management, entitled Organizational Decision Making Models: Comparing and Contrasting to the Stinson Wellness Model, won the Best Research Publication in Journal Award from the International Academy of Business and Economics (Volume 14, Number 3, 2014).

We plan to continue to write papers about how the model can be used in business settings. So if you are interested watch for them.

CONTACT INFORMATION

David D. Stinson
www.stinsoneducation.com
stinsoneducation@gmail.com

REFERENCES

Aerts, D., Apostel, L., De Moor, B., Hellemans, S., Maex, E., Van Belle, H., et al. (1994). *World Views From fragmentation to integration.* Brussels: VUB Press.

Amabile, T., & Kramer, S. (2011). *The Progress Principle: Using Small Wins to Ignite Joy, Engagement, and Creativity at Work.* Boston, Mass: Harvard Business Review Press.

Archer, J., Probert, B. S., & Gage, L. (1987). College students' attitudes to ward wellness. *Journal of College Student Personnel* , 28 (4), 311-317.

Bingle, G. (n.d.). Under the Sign of the Body: Naturalising Technological Well-Being in the Design of Wellness Users. Retrieved 8 5, 2004, from http://www.lrz-muenchen.de/~designing-the-user/papers/GBshotpaper.pdf.

Canadian Centre for Occupational Health and Safety (2015). Health & Wellness, retrived May 21, 2015; http://www.ccohs.ca/topics/well ness/.

Chickering, A. W. (1990). Education and Identity. San Francisco, California: Jossey-Bass Publishers.

Covey, S. R. (2004). The 8th Habit: From Effectiveness to Greatness. New York, New York: Free Press.

Deci, E. L., Ryan, R. M. (2008). Hedonia, Eudaimonia, and Wellbeing: an Introduction. *Journal of Happiness Studies, 9, 1-11.*

Diener, E., Wirtz, D., Tov, W., Kim-Prieto, C., Choi D., Oishi, S., Biswas-Diener, R. (2009). New Well-being Measures: Short Scales to Assess Flourishing and Positive and Negative Feelings. Springer Science+Business Media B. V., 143-156.

Dunn, H. L. (1961). *High Level Wellness.* Arlington, VA: R. W. Beatty, Ltd.

Dweck, C. S. (2007). *Mindset: the new psychology of success.* New York, New York: Ballantine Books.

Frankl, V. E. (1959). *Man's Search For Meaning.* New York, New York: Washington Square Press.

Grisham, J. (2000). *A Painted House.* New York, New York: Bantam Dell.

Hettler, B. (1998, September 25). *The Past of Wellness.* Retrieved June 27, 2013, from hettler.com: http://www.hettler.com/History/hettler.htm

Holmes, A. F. (1983). *Contours of a Worldview.* Grand Rapids, Michigan: William B. Eerdmans Publishing Company.

Horx, M. (n.d.). Was ist Wellness? Anatomie und Zukunftsperspektiven des Wohlfuh-Trends , n.p.

Illing, K. (1999). Der Gesundheitstourismus. Wellnes als Alternative zur traditionellen Kur?

Jung, C. J. (1933). *Modern man in search of a soul.* New York, New York: Harcourt Brace.

Keyes, C. L. M., Annas, J. (2009). Feeling good and functioning well: distinctive concepts in ancient philosophy and contemporary science. *The Journal of Positive Psychology*, 4, (3), 197-201.

Larson, D. D. (1999). The conceptualization of health. *Medical Care Research and Review* , 56, 123-136.

Leider, R. J. (1997). The Power of Purpose. San Francisco, CA: Berrett-Koehler Publishers.

Lucado, M. (2005). *Cure For The Common Life: Living in Your Sweet Spot*. Nashville, Tennessee: W Publishing Group.

Miller, J. W. (2005). Wellness: The History and Development of a Concept. *Spektrum Freizeit*, 1, 84-102.

Myers, J. E. (1992). Wellness, Prevention, Development: The Cornerstone of the Profession. *Journal of Counseling and Development*, 71, (2) 136-139.

Myers, J. E., & Sweeney, T. J. (2005). The Indivisible Self: An Evidence-Based Model of Wellness. *Journal of Individual Psychology*, 61 (3), 269-279.

Myers, J. E., & Williard, K. (2003). Integrating Spirituality Into Counselor Preparation: A Develepmental, Wellness Approach. *Counseling and Values*, 47, 142-155.

Myers, J. E., Sweeney, T. J., & Witmer, J. M. (2000). The wheel of wellness, counseling for wellness: A holistic model for treatment planning. *Journal of Counseling & Development*, 78, 251-266.

Norris, J. M., Williams, P.; O'Connor, M.; Robinson, J. (2013). An applied framework for Positive Education. *International Journal of Wellbeing*,

3 (2), 147-161.

Palmer, P. J. (2000). *Let Your Life Speak: Listening for the voice of vocation.* San Francisco, California: Jossey-Bass.

Pearcey, N. R. (2005). *Total Truth: Liberating Christianity from Its Cultural Captivity.* Wheaton, Illinois: Crossway Books.

Richardson, F. S. (2010). *"Lift up your voice" listening to elders in residential care and assisted living an action research study (doctoral dissertation).* Pomona, CA: Western University of Health Sciences, xvii, 178 p.

Rogers, C. R. (1961). On Becoming a Person. Boston: Houghton Mifflin.

Saxe, J. G. (1873). *The Poems of John Godfrey Saxe.* Boston, Massachusetts: James R. Osgood and Company.

Senge, P. M. (1990). *The Fifth Discipline: The Art & Practice of The Learning Organization.* New York, New York: Doubleday.

Shakespeare, W. (2008). *As You Like It.* Waiheke Island.

Sire, J. W. (2004). *Naming the Elephant: Worldview as a Concept.* Downers Grove, Illinois: InterVarsity.

Smith, B. J., Tang, K. C., & Nutbeam, D. (2006, September 7). *WHO Health Promotion Glossary: new terms.* Health Promotion International Advance Access , 5.

Travis, J., & Ryan, R. (1981, 1988, 2004). *Wellness Workbook.* Berkeley, CA: Ten Speed Press.

Waterman, A. S., Schwartz, S. J., Conti, R. (2008). The implications of two conceptions of happiness (hedonic enjoyment and eudaimonia) for the understanding of intrinsic motivation. *Journal of Happiness*

Studies, 9, 41-79.

Woolf, H. B. (Ed.). (1980). *New Collegiate Dictionary*. Toronto, Ontario: Thomas Allen & Son Limited.

World Health Organization (1958). *Constitution of the World Health Organization*. Retrieved 7 31, 2008, from World Health Organization: http://.who.int/governance/eb/who_constitution_en.pdf

World Health Organization (1986), *The Ottawa Charter for Health Promotion: First*
International Conference on Health Promotion, Ottawa, 21 November 1986, retrieved May 19, 2015, http://www.who.int/healthpromotion/conferences/previous/ottawa/en/.

World Health Organization, Health and Welfare Canada, and Canadian Public Health Association (1986). *Ottawa Charter for Health Promotion: An International Conference on Health Promotion--The Move To wards a New Public Health, Nov. 17-21, Ottawa* Geneva, Switzerland: World Health Organization.

Young, W. P. (2007). *The Shack*. Newbury Park,, California: Windblown Media.

CPSIA information can be obtained
at www.ICGtesting.com
Printed in the USA
BVHW032321120121
597634BV00003B/9